D0849856

The Culture of Biomedicine

The Culture of Biomedicine

Studies in Science and Culture, Volume 1

D. Heyward Brock, Editor
Ann Harward, Assistant Editor
Center for Science and Culture
University of Delaware

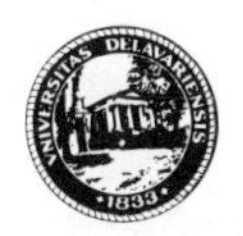

Newark: University of Delaware Press
London and Toronto: Associated University Presses

Associated University Presses, Inc.
440 Forsgate Drive
Cranbury, NJ 08512

Associated University Presses Ltd
25 Sicilian Avenue
London WC1A 2QH, England

Associated University Presses
2133 Royal Windsor Drive
Unit 1
Mississauga, Ontario L5J 1K5, Canada

Library of Congress Cataloging in Publication Data
Main entry under title:

The Culture of biomedicine.

(Studies in science and culture ; v. 1)
Contents: Science and humanities / Michael S. Gregory
—The goals of medicine and society / David C. Thomasma
—The phenomenon of medicine / Richard M. Zaner—
[etc.]
1. Medicine—Philosophy—Addresses, essays,
lectures. 2. Medicine and the humanities—Addresses,
essays, lectures. 3. Social medicine—Addresses, essays,
lectures. 4. Medical anthropology—Addresses, essays,
lectures. I. Brock, D. Heyward (Dewey Hayward),
1941– . II. Harward, Ann. III. Series.
[DNLM: 1. Philosophy, Medical. 2. Medicine in
literature. 3. Physician-patient relations. 4. Culture.
W 61 C9677]
R723.C838 1983 610′.1′9 83-40438
ISBN 0-87413-229-0

Printed in the United States of America

Contents

Preface

This is the first volume in an annual series sponsored by the Center for Science and Culture at the University of Delaware. Established in 1976, the center developed out of a grant from the National Endowment for the Humanities to support an instructional program in the Culture of Biomedicine emphasizing the historical, political, ethical, and cultural dimensions of biomedicine. Although since its founding the center has expanded its interests beyond biomedicine, it seemed appropriate that this first volume should focus on biomedicine, to which the center traces its roots.

In keeping with the center's instructional and research philosophy, each of the eleven essays provides an interdisciplinary perspective on the topic under consideration. Although each essay is discrete and complete in itself, the eleven essays may be roughly grouped, respectively, into five broad but not mutually exclusive subjects: an interdisciplinary worldview; the philosophy of medicine; scientific concepts of human nature; cultural aspects of patient treatment; and literature and medicine.

Although not focused on biomedicine, Michael Gregory's essay provides an orientation to, and a rationale for, an interdisciplinary worldview that integrates both the sciences and the humanities in a combined effort to illuminate human nature. Indeed, this essay may well serve as a general orientation to the interdisciplinary approach taken in the entire volume.

Analyzing the real and professed goals of both medicine and society, David Thomasma argues that health is a condition of well-being, a necessary condition, and an absolute value for human beings. He contends that "restoring health as the appropriate goal of medicine at once requires a moral analysis of the medical enterprise, an existential understanding of personal impairment, the relation of this impairment to other values, and an ordering of action according to these rational analyses." In his discussion of the phenomenon of medicine,

Richard Zaner explores the philosophical significance of the human body for the explanatory interests of medicine.

James Trosko describes some salient scientific concepts of human nature and assesses the various ethical implications of these concepts for technological intervention, emphasizing that "the purpose of explicating the scientific facts and theories of human nature . . . is to have all of us become sensitive to the alternative values that maximize individual potential and social responsibility, while at the same time avoiding values that tend irreversibly to tip that balance." Michael Ruse's detailed analysis of the evidence for and against taking sociobiology seriously as a scientific theory focuses on human sexuality and concludes that sociobiology has a long way to go before it can lay claim to being an established paradigm. More concerned about the realistic prospect for human survival than the cogency of scientific theories, Van Rensselaer Potter argues strongly for a bioethical creed that will lead to guidelines, laws, and actions that will help ensure the acceptable survival of future generations.

The essay by Coggins and Graham demonstrates the importance of understanding the cultural orientation of patients in effective treatment, and Dennis Carlson explains how drama and art can be utilized to improve the general health and quality of life for certain kinds of patients.

The last three essays deal with literature and medicine. Peter Graham explicates E. A. Robinson's poetic and delicate treatment of the controversial subject of euthanasia. Edmund Erde examines three films about physicians and healers, concentrating on how these works tend to reflect the essence of medicine in terms of pathos or pathology. Using literature as a mirror of humanity, Kathryn Rabuzzi challenges the concept of personality integration and argues that we may be witnessing the evolution of a new concept of human selfhood.

The subjects discussed and themes developed in these essays should provide the reader with a perceptive interdisciplinary overview of some of the most important aspects of the culture of biomedicine as it is understood in our day by many of those scholars most knowledgeable about the field.

D. HEYWARD BROCK

The Culture of Biomedicine

Science and Humanities: Toward a New Worldview

MICHAEL S. GREGORY

San Francisco State University

At a recent conference of scientists and humanists,[1] the principal topic of discussion was the question "Why do the sciences and the humanities need each other?" The presupposition was that these two great divisions of knowledge are capable of existing separately, which of course has been the case for at least three generations. But the question also presupposed that these domains of knowledge are in some important way incomplete in themselves and could gain by closer contact and better communication between them. As it turned out, that was indeed the consensus of the participants, who represented such broadly diverse fields as philosophy, literature, psychology, physics, biology, chemistry, and mathematics.

While the natural sciences have provided us with an astonishing amount of information about the world, they have told us little if anything about ourselves, and the humanities have done next to nothing to relate the world as given by science to us as human beings. Thus there is a void between the sciences and the humanities, and most of us live in that void. One of the purposes of this essay is to find ways to bring into focus information from the sciences and the humanities, and to argue that the point of that focus ought to be the human being.

I contend in this discussion that the human being as such is perhaps less well understood today than 100 or 300 years ago. We have more information but we understand less. One reason why this is so is that we have poorer, and less inclusive, hypotheses about human nature with which to conduct our thinking. These hypotheses, for the most part, fall under the heading of what I call "scientism." Scientism is a false synthesis, a pseudo-convergence, between the sciences and the humanities that has caused many problems. Scientism misrepresents the two domains to each other. It appears to answer questions but actually obscures them. Most important, scientism creates the illusion that the void between the sciences and the humanities has been abolished, that the two cultures have somehow been reunited, when in fact they have not.

Inasmuch as the materials of scientism are derived from science and received by humanities, it may appear that I am criticizing science itself. That is not the case. My criticisms are directed against the misappropriation and misuse of scientific information and the naive acceptance of such distorted information by both the humanities and the general public. In short, my argument is not with the Charles Darwins of this world, but with the Herbert Spencers—who are, sadly, with us still and in greater numbers.

My wish is that the sciences and the humanities may eventually come truly to know each other. In order for that to happen, some unproductive scientistic illusions need to be dispelled. If we can accomplish this, then the sciences and the humanities may be able to combine, on a firmer basis and on a broader front, to derive a genuinely humane study of human beings and their relation to the natural world. That is one reason, I think, why the sciences and the humanities need each other.

It is no news that humanities today are on the defensive. They have been, in fact, on the defensive for over a century, since the nearly simultaneous rise of the authority of science (accompanying and making possible the full flowering of the Industrial Revolution) and the decline of the authority of established religion. The decline of religion as an institution in the latter half of the nineteenth century was precipitate, like the sinking of the *Titanic.* If one must identify one particular iceberg, then it probably was Darwin's *Origin of Species,* published in 1859. What is not generally understood, even today, is how much of what we call humanities was invested in and supported by established Christianity—how much humanistic cargo was lost when the great ship went down.

By the 1880s, science was entering its age of triumph over a demoralized humanism that had lost not only its metaphysical sanctions, but much of its social utility. In the year 1880, Thomas Henry Huxley, "Darwin's Bulldog," began dismantling classical humanism as the presiding model for British education. In his lecture entitled "Science and Culture," Huxley lauded the founding of Sir Josiah Mason's Scientific College because its curriculum was based upon science and the acquisition of technological skills. Huxley was pleased to see that "mere literary education and instruction" were to be excluded, because they would lead, he claimed, only to "the ordinary smattering of Latin and Greek."[2]

Three years later, Matthew Arnold, the champion of classical humanism, was already backing off and taking a conciliatory tone toward science education. In his lecture "Literature and Science," Arnold proclaimed that "there is, therefore, really no question between Professor Huxley and me as to whether knowing the great results of the modern scientific study of nature is not required as part of our culture, as well as knowing the products of literature and art."

Arnold concluded, however, with a restatement of his claim that the study of humane letters was a better choice than science for "the great majority of mankind, all who have not exceptional and overpowering aptitudes for the study of nature. . . ."[3] Arnold's argument from the negative was a weak one, and deserved to lose. Inadvertently, Arnold anticipated by more than two generations C. P. Snow's "Two Cultures" hypothesis. Further, he conceded that a gulf existed between not only science and humanities, but also among the capabilities of those who enter these fields. Science was reserved for those particularly favored, while humanistic studies were left to those possessed of a less special intelligence.

Without the metaphysical and moral sanctions of religion, humanistic studies could pose no real competition for a burgeoning science. Indeed, it is better to call much of it scientism rather than science, because in the public mind the reverence for science rapidly approached a kind of idolatry. No greater proof for the intrinsic validity of science could be found, it would seem, than the Industrial Revolution itself, even though much of the Industrial Revolution was the product of what we today call technology. That is, it was the work of tinkerers, rather than scientists as such.

Herbert Spencer would weave a scientistic web broad enough to encompass and explain the entire universe, together with all of human social and political history, by analogies with and extensions of Darwin's theory of evolution. Such "Social Darwinism," as propounded by Spencer and a host of lesser spokesmen, had the powerful effect of combining a popular scientism with a defense of the status quo, including accumulated wealth, denigration of the poor, and British military colonialism. Perhaps its strongest appeal was that it was founded on (or purported to be founded on) science and reason—as opposed, of course, to the superstitions of the now largely superseded and discredited doctrines of established religion.

Science triumphed in the nineteenth century by providing concrete and tangible answers to human questions: How can one provide rapid communications from one part of the country to another? Answer: by building a great network of railways. How can one promote industrial prosperity? Answer: by establishing giant factories to produce steel and textiles, which in turn can be shipped for profit to all corners of the world. The list could be endless, and to the average Briton (and soon the average American) science became the religion of prosperity and progress. By means of science, mankind could leave behind the darkness and confusion of earlier times and enter into a new world of hope and light, of perfection of the social machine, of improvement without limit and without human cost.

We have now come to realize, of course, that for every question answered by science, a new question is first raised and then begged. The fundamental error of scientism has been the assumption that the paradigm within which science operates—that is, theory, hypothesis, demonstration, and validation—is coterminous with reality, both nonhuman and human. It should be noted that scientists are not themselves often guilty of scientism; the best never are. Responsible scientists are aware that data derived from one domain of investigation cannot logically or legitimately be transferred to another domain of investigation. To take a twentieth-century example, the last thing Albert Einstein, the founder of the Theory of Relativity, can properly be called is a relativist. Einstein's theory was in fact antirelativistic since it posited a universal constant, namely the speed of light. This transfer of explanation from one field to another is a falsification of science, yet it happens all too often. The clue to why it happens is found in what Emile Durkheim, the father of sociology, called a "social fact." A social fact may be demonstrably untrue in substance, but if it is believed by large numbers of people, it becomes true in a social sense. The notion of "ethical relativity" is an example of Durkheim's "social facts," insofar as people believe somehow that this brand of ethics is related to the Einsteinian hypothesis about space, time, and motion. Social Darwinism, which extended Darwin's hypothesis about biological processes into the realm of social processes, is probably the most flagrant example of a social fact used for vicious purposes.

To return to the main point: in the second half of the twentieth century, we are learning with increasing urgency that the questions answered by science are not always, or even often, the questions we as human beings need most to have answered. We are now coming to realize that questions that do not admit of scientific answers may nonetheless be valid questions to ask. Not many decades ago, it was commonly believed ("social fact") that if a question did not admit of being formulated scientifically, it was a nonquestion—an absurdity. We have had to undergo some period of disillusionment about the all-encompassing power of scientific explanation before we have been able to realize that such questions retain their qualitative validity and force for human beings. This creative disillusionment with scientism is best summed up by Lewis Thomas, author of *The Lives of a Cell.* "One way of looking at nature," Thomas tells us,

> is to put together all the facts learned thus far from the scientific revolution of this century, and to conclude that now is the time to make sense out of this information. If you do this, you are likely to agree with the current view in highest fashion, that making sense of nature is really no great problem. In this view, the ultimate answer, if you're so naive as to go looking for ultimate answers, is that it simply makes no sense, no sense at all. The world is meaningless. We are here through the blind accident of an infinite series of absolute random events. The sky is never blue; that is an optical illusion—the sky is black. The creatures of the earth are in endless conflict with each other, each hellbent on edging any nearby neighbor off the planet. Genes are the ultimate competitors

> and the sole survivors; tiny mindless strands of polymer are at the center of life. Man's place in nature is absurd. . . . The central, essential, existential dogma is that the universe is an insensate contraption, and we are caught, trapped in it. In the circumstance, we have no responsibilities except to our individual selves, and to the genes that invent those selves.[4]

Thomas goes on to say that such beliefs about the universe, and man's place in it, are no more than contemporary dogmas—what we have been calling here *scientism*—drawn from the data of cosmology, biology, and sociobiology, and put together as a philosophical worldview. Thomas himself believes that we have only begun to learn the secrets of nature, and that it is entirely premature, and even dangerous, to extrapolate from what we do know to what can ultimately be known. As Thomas wisely remarks, "Personally, if I could manage it, I'd rather stick around a while longer, around five centuries, say, and then see how it looks."

But it is clear that Thomas thinks that data from contemporary science are being misused, specifically to serve as the basis for a nihilistic view of the world. We should be especially concerned, consequently, with the process by which these "facts" have been transformed into "social facts," interpenetrating and mutually reinforcing. The process is one by which a contemporary worldview has been formed. Admittedly, this worldview is not much to write home about, but it is important to recognize that it is, indeed, a worldview, and that a good many people are using it, consciously or unconsciously, to justify, or to lament, their lives.

What above all is evident in this process is something that one may call *the drive for worldview.* As the French discovered in the aftermath of the Enlightenment, man lives not by reason alone, nor does woman either. Plainly put, human beings cannot survive on facts, especially disparate and limited facts emanating from separate domains of knowledge. The urge to put things together, whether they belong together or not, to forge from facts a system of thought and belief about the self and the world, is probably innate in our species. The problem is that worldviews are constructed as much from human aspirations, hopes, and needs as they are from observational data. Worldviews are not themselves scientific, although they may (as we have just seen) incorporate facts that individually may be corroborated scientifically. What we in the twentieth century have been painfully slow to recognize is that science and worldview cannot be exactly commensurate, even though each may contribute its share to the whole of human experience—but in very different ways.

What has happened in the last 100 years, however, is that science (for the most part inadvertently) smashed belief, not only invalidating the particular worldview of established Christianity, but invalidating the very notion of any nonscientific worldview whatever. It is pathetic to note that the human penchant for worldview, any worldview, survives, only now this worldview is structured from fragments of various scientific theories. One can only wonder what the shape of our worldview may be in ten or twenty years, when the information revealed by sociobiology is "borrowed" and incorporated into it.

By broad contrast, the classical Greek worldview was human-centered: the behavior of human nature was controlled by gods who resembled actual human beings (quarrelsome, loving, covetous, jealous, heroic) in every respect save only immortality. In effect, the Greeks demanded that the universe have human meaning and dimension. During the present century, however, we have completely reversed the process: we will admit as human only those aspects of ourselves that seem to be reflected in physical laws or biochemical processes or the behavior of lower life forms, most lately social insects. Our worldview, derived from misunderstood and misappropriated scientific information, fixes us as objects, rather than subjects, within a cosmos governed by randomness and uncertainty.

But we should take heart. Thomas, the philosophical medical researcher, like the poetic anthropologist Loren Eiseley, recognizes the essential uniqueness of *human* experience and the fact that human experience cannot be understood, let alone dealt with, on the basis of reductionism or analogy with processes that take place in other domains or on other levels of observation. Human beings must be taken in their own terms: not as congeries of atoms, or perceptual apparatus, or as machines for the reproduction of DNA. Thomas's article probably could not have been written twenty or even ten years earlier. We would not have been ready for it. He begins and ends with a premise that would have a generation ago provoked wry grins among social scientists and some humanists. The premise is that we are mysterious creatures, elusive to science, for better or worse inexplicably and unpredictably human. The human mind is as indeterminate as is the orbit of an electron, and we ourselves, the propounders of enigmas about the nature of the universe, are in fact the single greatest enigma in that universe.

We are still, in Matthew Arnold's famous phrase, "Between two worlds, one dying and the other powerless to be born." Actually, it is *two* worlds that are moribund, and a *third* that is struggling to be born. It seems altogether unlikely that very many of us can return to the comforting worldview of a Genesis literally accepted in each of its particulars. But it also seems unlikely, and increasingly so, that we will be able to persevere in a worldview in which we not only worship blindly a universal scientism, but reduce our conception of ourselves to fit only those processes that can be borrowed from scientific description. In this respect, Gerald Holton has recently written an account of the new field of sociobiology that serves as a paradigm for much of twentieth-century science. In his essay in *Sociobiology and Human Nature,* Holton writes:

> . . . Wilson's *Sociobiology* and related writings . . . may be viewed as significant cultural artifacts in their own right, because they represent a world view characterizing this part of the twentieth century—for example, in their plea for a sophisticated form of flexible, almost stochastic, predeterminism and materialism; in their apparently dispassionate concern with a secularized ethic; in their accent on rationality and their underemphasis on affect and symbolic forms. In short, with all their limitations, they exemplify what is widely considered to be some of the best thinking today.[5]

Holton continues with a plea for critical attention to the ethical and value implications of a modern materialist-mechanist reductionism such as that presented by the theories of sociobiology. It seems clear that Holton's plea is being heard, because sociobiology has been thrown on the defensive by concerted and well-planned counterattacks by philosophers, ethologists, and anthropologists. What is additionally significant is that an alliance among disciplines such as these would have been implausible, if not impossible, even a decade ago. The second world, the world of counter-Genesis, is also showing signs of reaching its limits. Please understand that I am not predicting the decline of science itself, but only of its misuse. I take it that this decline will be welcome to scientists and humanists alike.

It is easier to say what a new view of the world will *not* be than what it *will.* It will not be based exclusively upon quantification and measurement. It will not be bound by reductionistic principles under which, for example, the biological definition of a term such as *altruism* is derived from anthropomorphized descriptions of lower animals, nor will theories of cognition and communication be based upon assumed primate precursors.

In case that raises some eyebrows, consider the following fact, which has long been scanted: there is no more reason to believe that primate behavior is the evolutionary precursor of human behavior than there was, a hundred years ago, to assume that behavior among the Aranda of Australia is the evolutionary precursor of the behavior of European man. The error of logic is more readily spotted in the latter instance, because anthropologists have taught us that the Aranda's cultural evolution has as long a history as our own, but that it took a direction different from ours. There is, in logic, literally no better reason for believing that the chimpanzee's behavior patterns are the precursors of our own. The chimp has been around at least as long as we have, but he has met the conditions of his existence in different ways. The phylogenetic evidence simply will not allow the chimp to be our living ancestor, a fact that the chimpanzee, at least, would probably applaud.

Another thing one can say about the new worldview is that it will almost certainly not be based upon competition as the ultimate sanction. This use of competition was heavily overdone even in Darwin's initial formulation of natural selection, as Alfred Russell Wallace, the codiscoverer of evolution, pointed out in his later writings. During the past century, field observations corroborate the importance of cooperative, mutually supportive behavior not only within species, but among species. Prince Kropotkin's observations of Siberian wolves made the strong first case for cooperation, and more lately Desmond Morris has compiled a body of persuasive evidence for the lesser role of competition in group survival.

Yet another element in our current patchwork worldview is likely not to be found in the one that is emerging, and that is the scientistic legacy of quantum mechanics in subatomic physics. As fascinating in their own rights as are such precepts as the Heisenbergian uncertainty principle, in terms of which we can know the position or the velocity of an electron, but never both at the same time, and the corollary hypothesis that it is impossible to make an observation without disturbing the state of the thing observed, the picture they give us is of the interior world of the atom, and only that. Whether or not the structure of matter is governed solely by probabilities was a quarrel between Niels Bohr and Albert Einstein, and it has never been resolved. Nevertheless, the notion that the basic structure of matter is governed by chance, just as the Darwinian notion that change, in the form of spontaneous variations that govern the course of evolution, will almost certainly be seen as irrelevant and misleading as guides to the conduct of human affairs. "God does not play at dice with the world," said Einstein. While we have no direct knowledge of God's recreational habits, it is certainly safe to say that the behavior of subatomic particles has nothing whatever to do with whether we behave well or badly, morally or basely.

What lurks behind our current worldview is the need for uniformity and homogeneity at every level of explanation, and for every domain of phenomena: not only "As above, so below," but "As there, so here." Just as the prior, religious worldview achieved uniformity and homogeneity because of its assumed single source—that is, the mind of God—so the current worldview retains these same habits, although the sources are as divergent and incongruous as evolutionary biology and nuclear physics. The logical transfer from these fields to human cognition and epistemology is simply nil. In retrospect, one can only wonder at the need to "read" human beings in terms of the behavior of insects and electrons. The only reasonable explanation seems to be a hidden and silent need for a monistic, rather than pluralistic, view of the world, and one that is both hierarchically and laterally consistent. That may indeed be a property of all worldviews, including the patchwork one that is now reaching its culmination.

The worldview that is now beginning its struggle to be born will almost certainly have as its dominant characteristic the fact that it will again be human-centered, although not in quite so simplistic a way as was the worldview of the Greeks. We know too much, and perhaps too little, for that to occur again. One feature of this new worldview will be paramount: *human values for human beings.* If we are to understand ourselves within an evolutionary perspective, that perspective will not be prehuman biological evolution but the perspective of human cultural evolution, as Julian Huxley long ago predicted. We know next to nothing about cultural evolution, because it has never been the focus of sustained and systematic study. But we do know that for over one million years, man has adapted primarily by changing his *mind* (that is, his culture) rather than changing his *body.* The human world is one not of beaks and claws and fangs, but of ideas—although some of those ideas, admittedly, have been more lethal than any claw or fang. Again, we know next to nothing about the role of ideas in human cultures: how they arise, how they assume primacy within a group, how they conflict or combine, and how they change. We do know, however, that human ideas are almost infinitely variable, at least in that enduring form we call values. Values are ideas that have become part of a cultural tradition, an established worldview—so much a part that they tend to be transmitted unconsciously from generation to generation as part of the process of socialization. The term given by Alfred North Whitehead to such implicit values is "the general form of the forms of thought."

In 1933, Whitehead formulated a hypothesis about human values that ought to be part of the intellectual equipment of every philosopher and social historian, as well as of every anthropologist—indeed, of anyone wishing to understand the cognitive basis of human behavior. In his *Adventures of Ideas,* Whitehead presented the following theory of what might be called a *cultural unconscious* that silently shapes the thought of a particular culture at a particular point in its development. "In each age of the world distinguished by high activity," Whitehead writes,

> there will be found at its culmination, and among the agencies leading to that culmination, some profound cosmological outlook, implicitly accepted, impressing its own type on the current springs of action. This ultimate cosmology is only partly expressed, and the details of such expression issue into derivative specialized questions of violent controversy. The intellectual strife of an age is mainly concerned with these latter questions of secondary generality which conceal an agreement upon first principles almost too obvious to need expression, and almost too general to be capable of expression. *In each period there is a general form of the forms of thought; and, like the air we breathe, such a form is so translucent, and so pervad-*

ing, and so seemingly necessary, that only by extreme effort can we become aware of it.[6] [Emphasis added]

These "general forms" are cultural values, which lie beneath the level of awareness, which endure often for surprisingly long periods while undergoing sometimes startling surface transformations. In this regard, one thinks of China, which even under Mao retained the millennial imprint of Confucian values, such as benevolent paternalism, reference for scholarship, and Middle Kingdom cultural supremacy amid a barbarian world.

Values can be seen in a number of ways. Most superficially, they can be seen as conscious, shared judgments about what is good and bad, worthy and unworthy, laudable and despised. But, as Whitehead reminds us, such judgments are usually only the forms of thought, not the *form* of the forms, and therefore they are subject not only to rapid change, but to manipulation. Unfortunately, most of the current discussions about values center on what Whitehead called "questions of secondary generality." An example is pollution of the air by industrial smoke. At one time, and not long ago, it was a matter of pride for a community to be marked by a plume of smoke from its local factory. Indeed, World War II propaganda posters on both sides depicted homefront scenes of factories energetically belching smoke in the service of the war effort. That has changed dramatically, at least in the already developed countries. But what has not changed, or even been touched, at least until very recently, is the *form* of the forms—that is, the implicit value that the earth is here for the service of mankind and is to be exploited for mankind's exclusive benefit. The opposed implicit value—that the earth is our mother or our ancestor, and that we do harm to it only at our own peril—is found in premodern and nonwestern worldviews, but not in ours.

For our purposes, the profound sense of values—what the anthropologists Clyde and Florence Kluckhohn called *value orientations*—is what we need to understand if we are to discuss profitably the question of worldview. The subject has been given various names: for example, Edward Sapir called it "unconscious system of meanings"; Ruth Benedict used the expression "unconscious canons of choice"; Robert Redfield used the simple but satisfactory term "worldview." But regardless of minor terminological variations, the subject is the same:

namely, the patterns of choice characteristic of a culture and sustained from generation to generation by child-rearing and other socialization practices. Normally, Sapir points out, these choices are so implicit that one is entirely unaware that one is making them and is equally unaware that alternatives are possible.

At the same time, the study of comparative culture reveals wide discrepancies among the choices made and traditionalized by various peoples at various times. Florence Kluckhohn suggests several key loci of values, at which points all cultures make implicit choices.[7] These loci include *human nature*, which can be variously valued as all the way from innately good to innately evil, with a full range of mixtures of mutable good and evil in between. Similarly, *nature* itself may be viewed as hostile or benign, capable of being propitiated or indifferent, and the *relation between mankind and nature* can range from subjugation *of* nature to subjugation *to* nature, with a middle-ground of reciprocation and harmony. Another obvious locus of value is *time:* a culture, such as our own, may devalue the past and even the present in favor of investing value in a millennialist future. Confucian China, by contrast, valued remote antiquity, the Age of Yao and Shun invoked by Confucius as a period of unparalleled virtue, in comparison with which even his own present was a degeneration.

As I said before, presently we seem to be caught between three worlds—rather than the two envisioned by Matthew Arnold—the first of which is dead, the second of which has already reached its fullest extension, and the third of which is, indeed, still powerless to be born. A look at the value orientations, or form of the forms of thought, of the first two may yield clues about the structure of the future worldview.

The established Christian value system is the easier one to examine because we have about a century's critical distance from which to survey it. The traditional Christian view of man is, of course, lapsarian—that is, Adam and Eve were created good, but endowed also with freedom of choice. They were tempted, committed sin, and fell. Under the doctrine of Original Sin, therefore, mankind is evil but redeemable. Christianity adds a more immediate form of redemption via the vicarious atonement of Christ's passion on the cross, but humankind remains inherently debased, although capable of salvation.

Christianity's orientation toward time is distinctive, inasmuch as it is probably more thoroughly oriented toward the future (the Kingdom of God on Earth) than any other worldview that has ever existed. Indeed, it has been persuasively argued that the modern view of history—a beginning, a middle, and an end—would be impossible without the cognitive framework provided by Christian worldview. In this view, the thrust is ever toward the future; the past is shame, the present is part of the long process of purgation, and the end will be the destruction of the world and the coming of the Kingdom of God. It is this orientation toward the future, with its accompanying devaluation of both past and present, that survives to give Western culture its characteristic thrust. This thrust has, over the centuries, been both secularized and radically revised into the lay notion of progress. The idea of progress is unique to Western culture and imparts to it a dynamism that is both envied and feared by other cultures.

In Judeo-Christian tradition, mankind's relation to the earth is at one of the two furthest extremes in the record of human value orientations. In Genesis, God exhorts Adam to "go forth and subdue the earth." The earth, then, is by extension an inexhaustible resource, in itself devoid of value, to be used by human beings in whatever manner they see fit. In this tradition, which of course still survives in secularized form, there is no kinship or interdependence between mankind and the earth. Other traditions, by contrast, see the earth as the mother of life, to be tended and cherished. Ch'an (Zen) Buddhism, for example, together with Taoism, sees no subject-object distinction between human and other life, or between life itself and the interactive constituents of nature. The Ch'an precept of *wu-wei* (literally, "doing nothing") is the extreme opposite of our own in the record of human value orientations. Most cultures see the relationship between human and the world as reciprocally dependent. Our own tradition looks extremely odd, by the way, when viewed from the outside.

The worldview that presently obtains in the West continues the secularized features of Judeo-Christian tradition: future orientation in the form of progress and conception of the earth and its resources as mankind's inexhaustible playground. But, curiously, it drops the essential feature of the older tradition, namely the inherent evil of mankind. In a sense, the modern view of man does him even less honor, since it denies to him the capacity for either good or evil. Indeed, it denies to him the stature of human being, in the sense of possessing capabilities of awareness, choice, and will. The best description of the current worldview is that given by Gerald Holton, cited earlier: "Predeterminism and materialism . . . dispassionate concern with a secularized ethic . . . accent on rationality and . . . underemphasis on affect and symbolic forms." If one takes sociobiology seriously (and one had better take it seriously), the very conception of a human being is impossible. As Richard Dawkins explains in *The Selfish Gene*:

> Individuals are not stable things; they are fleeting. Chromosomes, too, are shuffled into oblivion, like hands of cards soon after they are dealt. But the cards themselves survive the shuffling. The cards are the genes. The genes are not destroyed by crossing over; they merely change partners and march on. That is their business. They are the replicators, and we are their survival machines. When we have served our purpose, we are cast aside. But genes are denizens of geological time: Genes are forever.[8]

To this one must add that the sociobiological hypothesis centers on the genetic coding, not merely of morphological characteristics, but of patterns of behavior, modes of consciousness, and, of course, values themselves. The sociobiological explanation of human nature (E. O. Wilson's latest book is entitled *On Human Nature*, and it was a Book-of-the-Month Club selection) is now in the ascendant. One hopes that its career will be short, because it is without doubt the most extreme reductionism ever applied to an explanation of human nature, and it contains within it some exceptionally dangerous ideas—potentially far more dangerous than the Social Darwinism that led to, among other things, Hitler's racial policies—because they emanate not from a popularizer like Herbert Spencer but from an eminent biologist like Wilson of Harvard. The notion that human values are shaped by genes would reduce human nature to purely mechanistic predeterminism, and "values" themselves would become useless concepts, to be abandoned in favor of phylogenetically derived categories of reptilian-mammalian behavior. Humanities, incidentally, would literally be reduced by Wilson to the status of research protocols on a single species, *Homo sapiens*. But humanities would be in good company, because both social science and conventional biology would be subsumed under a single discipline—namely sociobiology.[9]

The primary characteristics, then, of the contemporary

worldview are the following: quantities rather than qualities; probabilities rather than principles; mechanistic forces rather than states of being; and, above all, molecular rather than molar explanations of complex events. This is reductionism, the assumption that what holds true at lower levels of organization must also hold true at higher levels of organization.

Thus, the contemporary worldview is very much based upon discoveries about the smallest units of heredity, the gene, and about the smallest units of matter, the subatomic particle. These discoveries are then read upward to explain the behavior of human beings as individuals and as groups, and indeed the nature of the universe in general. The face that the argument is logically false does not matter; in fact, biologists such as Wilson argue for the productivity of reductionism, while ignoring the fact that it is logically untenable. The modern penchant for reductionistic explanations may have the function, oddly enough, of making people feel themselves as being part of the world—even a world that is governed by activity evident only at the lowest conceivable levels of analysis. If this is true, then it is the exact reverse of the Judeo-Christian worldview, which was *de*ductionistic—that is, it began with what could be understood about the nature of God, and read these data downward to explain lower level events, including human behavior, but extending also to the biological sciences and geology. One of the most striking features of the history of human thought is its tendency to swing from one extreme to the other, only rarely pausing to strike a balance in the middle.

To strike a balance in the middle will almost certainly be a feature of the new worldview. Prophecy is a dangerous game, but I would be willing to risk a few guesses based upon what I observe to be the strains evident in the current, scientistic worldview. First, the world as given in this view is a cold, hostile, meaningless place, as Lewis Thomas observes. Second, it ignores the fact that even though human beings must exist in a material world that is structured by scientific principles (assuming present paradigms stand the test of time, as Lewis himself doubts), it is also true that human beings live in a world of their own making.

For example, the most striking contribution made by Existentialism is the proposition that we can and do make our own ontological world, even if it is inconsistent with respect to the workings of the nonhuman universe. The willingness to accept this inconsistency, to break with the ancient imperative, "As above, so below," is probably a permanent contribution of Existentialism to a new form of humanism. Added to that is the contribution of a few psychologists and anthropologists, notably Frank Beach and Marshall Sahlins, warning against the modern reductionistic imperative, "As below, so above."

The new worldview, I venture to guess, will make an equal break with the past and with the present. It will not seek supernatural sanctions for human values, nor will it seek what Wilson calls "morality of the gene," nor attempt to make moral philosophy out of the behavior of electrons or pi-mesons. I should hope that the new worldview will manage to avoid such *post hoc* deadends. Simply because the genetic code or the physical structure of matter is anterior to the development of the human being does not mean that the human being can be explained by these means.

What has brought us to our present impasse is an abuse of both rational and intuitive modes of thinking. We have already discussed the rational abuses, principally the extension of the scope of explanation from one domain of knowledge to another, usually in the form of reductionistic analogies. But the intuitive abuses are just as marked. Probably the greatest human need, and it is thoroughly nonrational, is to feel at home in the universe. Why this should be so, I do not know. But human beings seem to reject energetically any notion that they and the universe into which they have been born are constructed according to different principles. It is for this reason, I think, that the cold, indifferent, and essentially meaningless picture of the universe as revealed by contemporary science has, at great human cost, been embraced as a "social fact" within our contemporary worldview. It is as if, faced with a choice between belonging nowhere and belonging in a prison, mankind has accepted the prison.

I think it is already becoming clear that we are capable of living, and even thriving, in a discontinuous universe: that is, a universe structured below according to microbiological and biochemical principles, a universe structured both within and above according to the principles of physics, but also a universe at our own level that is constructed according to human principles. I do not mean to espouse Luddite belief, by means of which we would simply ignore the data of science and be proud of our ignorance. Far from it. What I am suggesting is that we learn to live with conceptual asymmetry, and no longer insist, like children, that systems of explanation be the same on every level of phenomena. I am also suggesting that we get back to the work of being human, that we approach the dimensions of our humanness with the same zeal and wonder and productivity that we have lavished on molecular biology and particle physics. As Lewis Thomas says, "Our part in the world is unfathomable because we have not learned enough, but it is surely not absurd. We have some kind of importance here, for all our bewilderment. We are a significant part of the System. What we do with ourselves, and with the rest of life, makes a difference."

Let me give, in closing, a few examples of the cultural loci where new kinds of values may well be already appearing, as part of the birth of a new and more inclusive worldview. First is creativity. We ought really to accept the fact that human creativity is just about impossible to understand within any of the existing scientific models of explanation. I know about Kohler's chimps and the Japanese macaque monkey that invented rice-washing and snowball rolling. I also know about Koko and her ability to acquire and to manipulate sign language. I am aware of these examples, and I am not overwhelmed. They no more resemble the human creative process than a glowworm resembles the planet Venus. For spectacular examples of human creativity, of complex ideas springing apparently *ex nihilo,* I wish to recommend Arthur Koestler's excellent study, *The Act of Creation.*[10] It is stupefying to realize that this characteristic, that truly distinguishes us from everything else in the universe—that is, our ability to create entirely new ideas, forms, and methods—has gone almost wholly neglected as an object of study during this century.

Second is culture. Animals, even and especially insects, form societies, but only mankind forms cultures. Culture, as a body of learned behavior, rather than a preprogrammed body of drives and instincts, is as unique in the universe as creativity—indeed, it may be the most outstanding example of creativity among human beings. Since culture is learned, it allows for rapid modification, especially when such modification is necessary for survival. Consider again, mankind adapts, not by changing its bodily form, but by changing its mind. As David Barash has observed, biological evolution is Darwinian, while cultural evolution is Lamarckian. The cognitive aspects of culture have gone almost entirely neglected within recent years, yet an understanding of cultural consciousness seems essential to an understanding of our human modes of conceptualizing the world and dealing with one another. One of the most striking features of culture—and this is the hallmark of distinctive human activity in general—is its almost limitless variety and the uniqueness of each cultural configuration.

Third is language. For two generations, we have sought to understand language on the basis of signaling practiced by the lower animals or, following Chomsky, on the basis of some presumably inherited deep structure, corresponding to the evolution of the brain. But such deterministic studies tend to minimize or ignore the spontaneity of language and the capacity of language to convey entirely fresh meanings, nuances, and affective states. The work of Sapir, Whorf, and Lee, in which language was seen as shaping the mode and manner of cognition, continues to be fascinating. Indeed, their theories claimed that our conception of reality is structured by the particular syntactical and grammatical properties of the language we use. But still, these hypotheses scant what is probably the most salient and impressive characteristic of human language. That characteristic is, again, its capacity for novelty and unpredictability, and especially its capacity to convey complex emotive and intuitive states from one human speaker to another, to bring about empathy (from two Greek words meaning "to feel into" the thoughts and feelings of another person). The highest use of language, as well as the most powerful instrument for transferring innovative thought, is of course literature. But here again, literature has never been systematically studied from this point of view. The other arts, particularly music and painting, demand parallel kinds of attention as modes of conveying cognitive-affective-intuitive states from one mind to other minds.

Fourth and finally is self-directed behavior—what is commonly called morality. Man is the only animal capable of moral behavior, and perhaps the only animal that needs it. In philosophy, a distinction is made between ethics and morality, and it is important to observe that distinction here. Ethics are public values; they govern what one does or does not do when others are watching. Morals, on the other hand, are private values; they govern what one does or does not do when no one is watching. Strikingly direct parallels with human ethical behavior may be observed among animals. The famous "look" given by father baboon to baby baboon, even though they may be separated by fifty yards, is enough to make baby baboon cringe as before a blow and to cry out in real pain. Ethical behavior is enforced by outside sanctions, all the way from the "look" to punishment to the cruelest sanctions of all—ostracism and banishment.

Moral behavior uses no sanctions, for it requires none. It may be learned, as the Freudians postulate, but giving it a name like superego does not tell us much about its operation. There seems to be no good reason not to describe the moral sense in its most obvious form: that is, as a mental representation of the self to the self, a representation against which actual or contemplated behaviors can be measured and judged. Insofar as this representation is the product of socialization processes, the self may be thought of as the internal form of cultural values. But the particular blend and balance of these values, their cognitive shape and pattern, are highly individualized. As far as we know, the human being is the only animal that establishes such normative mental images of itself, maintains them through time, and makes choices on the basis of harmony or discord with such images. In a word, human beings are capable of character, which is a durable and consistent self-representation that serves as guide and corrective for personal action.

In the early years of this century, the psychologists William McDougall and William James attempted to found a scientific study of character. McDougall called this study "characterology," which probably was enough to doom it from the start. Among contemporary psychologists, it is fashionable to look upon this attempt to formulate theories of character as primitive, pre-Freudian, and pre-Jungian psychology. Yet McDougall and James were neither primitives nor fools. They wished to study human mental functioning in its largest and most comprehensive aspects, rather than in the lesser psychological quanta that came to be known as neuroses, psychoses, and complexes. McDougall's and James' work fell to the anatomizing spirit of this century, and especially it fell to our overwhelming penchant for reductionism. For example, Freud believed he could trace the origin of artistic creativity to infantile fecal play. Jung mythologized about racial memories and inherited images—what he termed archetypes and imagos.

Neither the Freudian nor Jungian approach allowed for the apprehension of the fully developed, complex, multi-faceted phenomenon of character, so there is at this moment not even a term in the psychologist's handbook for character in the positive sense. The only term that exists is pejorative, and it is "character disorder." But if character is the behavioral expression of the moral sense, and if the moral sense is our capacity to form a consistent and durable mental image of a valued self, then morality and character are as distinctively human, and therefore as deserving of fresh attention, as creativity, language, and culture.

Each of these may be predicted to be a principal locus of value within the emerging worldview. These are reasonably safe predictions because they are key segments of any system of values that would center once more on human experience. This new worldview would be liberating, for several reasons. First, it would free us of the necessity of attempting to comprehend human experience in terms that are not only logically inappropriate but that also violate everything we intuitively know is essential to that experience. We are made up of genes and atoms, but that does not mean that our experience is reducible to genes and atoms, nor does it mean that our actions are bound by the same iron laws of determinism that they are.

We know intuitively that we are free, or at least are capable of being so. Why we have so long fled from this intuition is a major question for psychology and philosophy. Jean-Paul Sartre once observed that freedom is terrifying, and that many people unconsciously yearn to become inorganic things in order to escape the responsibility of being free. Mankind's political history seems repetitively to tell us the same thing, and Erich Fromm has written of the awesome burdens of individuality. But nothing in our accumulated knowledge about ourselves and our nature tells us conclusively that we are not free to be free. We do know that we are, inexplicably, strangers to the universe, and that its ways are not our ways, but that does not mean that we are less than human. There is apparently only one spot in the whole of the cosmos that is not irretrievably fixed by the laws of entropy and determinism, and that spot is the human mind. Loren Eiseley once defined the human brain as nature's single experiment with an organ of indeterminacy.[11] Nature took a chance on us, he says, and invented a being that manipulates time, that forms images of the future, that lives on dreams.[12]

In sum, perhaps we are finally ready to accept, among the swirl of atoms and random forces and the dying out of stars, the uniqueness of our species. Perhaps it will prove true, as Pierre Boulle has said, that *Homo sapiens* is the missing link between the animal and the human being.

NOTES

1. The NEXA/CSUC Dissemination Conference, June 19–20, 1980, Asilomar Conference Center, Pacific Grove, California. NEXA is a function of San Francisco State University and combines team-taught courses aimed at the convergence of sciences and humanities with public events programming and dissemination to other institutions. It is supported by the National Endowment for the Humanities, the Andrew W. Mellon Foundation, the California Council on the Humanities, and San Francisco State. It has received additional support for conferences from the chancellor of the California State University and Colleges (CSUC), the system of nineteen campuses of which San Francisco State University is a part. This essay is based upon a presentation made at the conference on June 20. Readers wishing to learn more about the NEXA program or to exchange ideas with members of its faculty are invited to write to the director, NEXA Program, School of Humanities, San Francisco State University, San Francisco, California 94132.

2. Thomas Henry Huxley, *Science and Culture and Other Essays* (1881). Reprinted as "Science and Culture" in *Science and Literature,* ed. John J. Cadden and Patrick K. Brostowin (Boston: D. C. Heath and Co., 1964), p. 11.

3. Matthew Arnold, *Discourses in America* (Lecture 2: "Literature and Science") (1883–84). Reprinted as "Literature and Science" in *Science and Literature,* p. 17.

4. Lewis Thomas, "The Strangeness of Nature," *New England Journal of Medicine* 298 (1978): 1454–55. Subsequent quotations from Thomas are from this source.

5. Gerald Holton, "The New Synthesis?" in *Sociobiology and Human Nature,* ed. Michael S. Gregory, Anita Silvers, and Diane Sutch (San Francisco, Calif.: Jossey-Bass, 1978), p. 79.

6. Alfred North Whitehead, *Adventures of Ideas* (New York: Macmillan Co., 1933). Republished as a Mentor Book (New York: New American Library of World Literature, 1955), pp. 19–20.

7. Florence Kluckhohn and Fred L. Strodtbeck, *Variations in Value Orientations* (Evanston, Ill.: Roe, Peterson and Co., 1961). The schema for value orientations is based upon that presented in this work.

8. Richard Dawkins, *The Selfish Gene* (New York and Oxford: Oxford University Press, 1976), p. 37.

9. If one thinks this is strong medicine, I recommend reading both of Wilson's books, *Sociobiology: The New Synthesis* (Cambridge, Mass.: Harvard University Press, 1975) and *On Human Nature* (Cambridge, Mass.: Harvard University Press, 1978), and as a corrective, a book entitled *Sociobiology and Human Nature* (see note 5 above), which contains criticisms of the new field from the perspectives of philosophy, anthropology, and ethology.

10. Arthur Koestler, *The Act of Creation* (New York: Macmillan Co., 1964). Republished as a Dell Laurel Edition (New York: Dell Publishing Co., 1967).

11. Loren C. Eiseley, *Darwin's Century* (New York: Doubleday and Co., 1958), pp. 349–52.

12. Loren C. Eiseley, "Fossil Man and Human Evolution," in *Current Anthropology*, ed. William L. Thomas (Chicago: University of Chicago Press, 1956), p. 68.

The Goals of Medicine and Society

DAVID C. THOMASMA

Loyola University of Chicago Medical Center

If our magazines, newspapers, and popular literature are valid thermometers of our culture, then the temperature of medicine is rising. During the past few years the number of articles on medical topics has exploded. *Esquire* magazine, for example, during 1976 carried some article or short story on a medical topic almost every month. In that year, articles, some by physicians, appeared on the twin doctors found dead in New York City, on the Janker clinic in Germany and the American Cancer Society, on baldness, on the body, on abortion, and on coronary bypass surgery.[1]

One might be tempted to think attention paid to medical topics by popular but serious publications arises from the fact that medicine now accounts for about 9 billion dollars of the yearly federal budget, the third largest expenditure. This figure does not include state and local expenditures, nor those of the private citizen.

In 1977, a March 29 American Medical Association publication cited an unpublished report by the Federal Wage and Price Stability Board showing that the average family spends more than a ninth of its income on health care. Each year medical insurance payments rise by more than 18 percent. By April 1980, health care costs far outstripped all other inflationary trends, even the increasing price of gasoline. Polls showed citizens unwilling to pay more even if they could be assured of increased quality.

No doubt the remarkable rise of interest in medical topics is related to its share of budgets. But there is a deeper reason. Medicine has become an expression of culture. Not only a preoccupation, medical topics represent an interest in an organizing principle of society, one block upon which we build our images of man and the future. One glibly speaks of healthy institutions, sick structures. Plans for a long life and old age are an intrinsic part of our self-image. Avoiding pain has become a predominate occupation of human beings. The goals of medicine and the aspirations of human beings in society appear on the surface to be working in harmonious tandem. Like a rotary engine smoothly churning out the future, society seems to provide the spark and medicine the torque. Society holds before us our own aspirations for the good life, and medicine seems to be increasing the possibility for that life. Surely there is nothing wrong with this picture.

But there is a note of trouble. The rotary engine seems a bit out of tune. Our first inkling comes when we are told that Preparation H contains a "soothing" ingredient recommended by "hemorrhoidal experts." Our awareness increases while subjected to the eternal debate about which pain reliever is best, or which one New York doctors recommend most, or even the one to which government studies attest. Awareness reaches a pinnacle during ads depicting a growling stomach, deodorant tampons (after all, what *does* she know that we don't?), whispered secrets about diarrhea, and so on. A conviction grows. Medicine is used to sell nonmedical ideals. Many of these products are only remotely related to authentic medical concerns.

If popular literature reflects our culture, then personal convictions are confirmed. At root there is a concern about life without wisdom, about living too long without some answers to the meaning of life. Just pick up a back issue of *Esquire* again. In the Bicentennial issue, short sketches of American lives reveal concerns about missing the point of life. For example, Nora Ephron wonders about a fur coat, a symbol of life that made no sense in her mother's death. In another issue, John Sack attacks a pediatrician because he was a social engineer. In a short story Sack writes of his own babyhood, the restrictions placed on feeding and touching, and the impact of these on his own life. His point is that every person is perfect and in loving unity with the cosmos. And then something—modern medicine—happens. Because of the influence of modern medical science, Sack accuses Americans of forming a model of man as a "reed, indeed, a thing that's made out of matchsticks that has to be glued and be guy-wired at ten thousand points or it topples apart."[2]

The forgoing suggests that the relationship between medicine and society, particularly as it affects a vision of man, is worth serious analysis. In the first section of this essay, I explore this relationship. My thesis is that medicine and society do interact to form a definition or picture of a human being. In the second section of the paper, I look at the professed and real goals of both medicine and society in this interaction. I close with a proposal for appropriate goals of medicine and society.

This is a difficult task. Any prediction of trends and the future is subject to the Harvard Law, which states: "Under the most rigorously controlled conditions of pressure, temperature, volume, humidity, and other variables, the organism will do as it damn well pleases."[3] There are too many medical and social variables to make definitive statements. Thus, this essay stands only as a plea for more qualitative discussion about the goals of medicine and society.

RELATION BETWEEN MEDICINE AND SOCIETY

A good place to start exploring this relationship might be to join Don DeLillo in a *Gedankexperiment*, a thought-experiment. Picture, as he does, a 150-year-old man, an aged scientist of the future turned mystic. Poetic license will allow alterations to his story. Let me call this man Grimes Posnovich. Grimes, at age 21, produced semen for storage in an SS bank (SS for Security Semen company). Unlike his other contemporaries, who also were sterilized but who were able to have six generations of direct descendants from their semen, Grimes was involved in a lawsuit when an equipment failure at the bank destroyed his reproductive abilities. Attempts to reverse the operation failed. He has waited in vain for his aged wife to be cloned, since difficulties have arisen in procedures. At 63, he received coronary bypass surgery. A Pacemaker was installed. No further difficulties have developed besides the usual problem of batteries. Later he had an artificial kidney implant (donated or-
ns from other animals), two cancer operations, and has been
cted to artificial food, processed to keep him alive at all
many senses, Grimes is a bionic man, like the popular

television character. But he is unable to leap tall buildings. Instead he lives in a bio-membrane machine, unable to communicate with younger members of society because of the rapid, geometrically changing conditions of life.

His machine is wheeled into the room, while he struggles to breathe. Three inhalation therapy aides hover around him at all times, like acolytes. He has not worked since age 55 and has spent the remaining 95 years of his life as a ward of the state, like so many of his contemporaries. Despite the use of happiness drugs, he is depressed because he does not feel productive or even self-determined.

According to DeLillo's story, Grimes's bio-membrane machine sports the following decals and looks like the racing machines of long ago:

> MAINLINE FILTRONIC
> Tank and Filter Maintenance
>
> STERILMASTER PEERLESS AIR CURTAINING
> The Breath You Take is the Life We Save
>
> BIZENE POLYTHENE COATING
> U.D.G.A. Inspected and Approved
>
> WALKER-ATKINSON METALLIZED UNDERSURFACES
> From the Friendly Folks at Uniplex Synthel
>
> EVALITE CHROME PANELING
> The Glamour Name in Surgical Supplies
>
> DREAMAWAY
> Bed Linen, Mattress, and Frame
> A Division of OmCo Research
> "Building a Model World"[4]

While this whimsical picture of Grimes Posnovich contains elements of tragedy, nothing described is beyond present-day medical science, or at least its presumed aim.[5] But note some significant changes in self, social, and medical images.

The *Gedankexperiment* about Grimes Posnovich leads to some important questions and observations. Because medicine and society interact on so many levels, consider only one goal of medicine, the prolongation of life. Increasing life expectancy to 150 years creates major changes in the self-image of man and society, which in turn has an impact on medicine. Bear in mind that I am touching on only a few factors of an even larger picture of man and technology; consequently, my observations are apt to be slightly over-simplified.

The direction of medicine toward life-prolongation leads to an increasingly positivistic view of man as a biologically functioning machine. Considered socially, our political system no longer preserves life in its fuller dimensions, but enhances only the biological quality of life. Already this is happening. Allocation of federal funds for biological research far exceeds allocations for the arts and humanities.[6] But preoccupation with the biological at the expense of qualitative factors of life is dangerous to the practice of medicine as well. Jerky, breathy, emphesemic attempts are made to treat the whole man, but inevitably fail. Why? First, they fail because focus upon biological life-prolongation leads to defining man in merely biological terms. Consequently, the whole man becomes an illusive fog. No one can tell what it means.[7]

Second, focus upon life-prolongation by using machines and life-support systems, like Grimes's bio-membrane capsule, leads to an image of man as increasingly dependent. The more dependent upon machines, drugs, and other artificial devices we become, the less self-determined we are. The freedom of man began to be questioned only in the age of the machine. If one views freedom as the ability to choose, to commit oneself, and to create new choices, one can see that all three are truncated in the case of Grimes Posnovich. He cannot move except when others move his capsule; he cannot choose his food because it has become standarized for his own good. He cannot commit his life to a meaningful goal. This lack of self-determination has a profound effect upon the political assumption that human beings are free. Social truncation of real freedom will inevitably result. Grimes has already become a ward of the state. Hence, there is more social control over his life, as well as over the medical treatment offered him. Medicine itself begins to suffer increased control by social forces, and not always for the good of those it serves.[8]

Third, Grimes's communicative abilities, including sexual [illegible]nes, have been severely limited. He can only speak over the [illegible]membrane. In a broader sense, any dependency decreases [illegible]bility to communicate, and communication must take [illegible]ugh the technological product. The medium becomes the message. The definition of man is profoundly influenced by modes of communication. While studies of the effect of computers and television on the self-definition of man remain incomplete, they at least suggest profound changes in our concepts of self and society. For example, some thinkers postulate that the invention of printing was a major cause of the Reformation because attention to the printed word of the Bible became more important than the larger pictorial approach of Roman Catholic art and architecture.

Pedro Lain-Entralgo, a Spanish philosopher of medicine, has examined the social impact of changing concepts of therapy of the word on changing concepts of medicine. It is probable that in Grimes's time, medicine will communicate through extremely overspecialized symbolism. One branch of medicine will barely be able to understand the other. This overspecialization will duplicate the same problem in society. Relationships will be seen only in an externalized fashion. Bits and pieces of man and of society will hinge together, as in Sack's view, like a matchstick. Fragmentation of man leads to fragmentation of society.

If relationships among things and people are only seen externally, as a political necessity, then social value-consensus decreases. Because value-consensus depends upon a discovery of inherent commonalities, its decrease will lead to burgeoning overload of court cases. In our society, when we profoundly disagree, we appeal finally to the courts. Losing any sense of being able to pose and even answer the larger questions about life, we will increasingly produce *ad hoc* solutions to problems, each one stumbling over the other.[9]

Is there any reason to believe that our steadily increasing tendency to ask only small questions and treat definable problems will decrease in the future? Is there any reason to believe that the lack of value-consensus will decrease our tendency to go to court? Look for incredible malpractice claims in the future.[10]

Fourth, the use of artificial devices to prolong life will lead to a vision of man as technological product. Most of us are not opposed to the use of artifice to help the suffering, but we should be aware of the changes in self-definition these pose. Ellul, Mumford, Dubos, and others have explored the change in man that comes about through dependency upon a technological system of our own creation. While their vision is negative, at least we can see that a mechanized view of man and society does result.

Among the many spin-offs of an overly mechanized view of man and society is the loss of flexibility, which has a profound result on medicine itself, and indeed, on all the professions. For the essence of a profession is the flexibility of judgment necessary for its exercise. Many physicians oppose the increase of court judgments and social intervention upon their professional judgments for precisely this reason. Once again I ask, is there any reason to assume that the dramatic increase of technology in medicine and society will lead to a decrease in a mechanized and rigid interpretation of life? Grimes Posnovich lives in a socially rigid society. The complex nature of his machine and the social and economic web that keep it functioning sacrifice flexibility for life-prolongation. Is that what human beings really want?

Finally, the life-prolonging goals of medicine will change the concept of work and leisure. Ironically, while society pushes us to retire early (Grimes retired at 55), it is also pushing life-prolongation. Just as ironically, the technology to effect life-prolongation, among other goals, demands of its workers a sense of productivity—hence, the definition of man as productive. Marx was eulogized by Engels at the graveside for his insight that man is by nature productive and that the meaning of man was found in work. If the true meaning of human existence for our time is found in productivity, then small wonder leisure time must also be productive. Americans are extremely busy about their leisure, and I see no signs that this value will decrease with our ability to prolong life. Imagine how difficult it will be to discover some other sense of human and social existence in Grimes's dependent role, if our own old people now feel like social garbage at worst, social decoration at best.

Robert P. Hudson, M.D., has brought to light another ironic feature of the dilemma of productivity. In 1962, a Seattle electrician who had not adequately provided for his family of six children was adjudged by two physicians, an attorney, a banker, a labor leader, and housewife, to be more productive than two other men, both better educated and better providers for their families. The electrician received a kidney transplant, while the other two died in a matter of weeks. Hudson believes that comfortable moral blinders will soon have to come off, the major one being that we really have a reverence for life. Instead, economic values and productivity are the standards by which many of our medical judgments are made.[11]

I add to Hudson's account a triple irony. Prolongation of life is based on a respect for life; the technological capacity for prolonging life depends upon increased productivity, upon productivity as the measure of a man. This value eventually leads to decisions based on productivity rather than reverence for life. The original reason for prolonging life—reverence for life—is destroyed. Which comes first, medical factors, social factors, or human self-definition? It might be best to say that the three interact upon one another.

What conclusion can be reached? While not exhausting all considerations possible in the *Gedankexperiment* about Grimes Posnovich, we can conclude at least that medicine and society do interact, although not always for the best. This interaction also involves human self-definition. The important factors of human life are a sense of wholeness, a sense of self-determination and freedom, a sense of community (at least a community of values), a sense of creativity, sexuality, and communication. In all of these areas, prolonging life contains seeds of destruction, not only of man's self-image, but also of medicine itself.

These reflections point out, I think, the danger of our present situation. If medicine begins filling the void left by the departure of religion, if the second half of the ancient term religious-medicine man gains dominance over the first half, then we are faced with what Ivan Illich calls the overmedicalization of society. Illich, with words revealing the danger, accuses medicine of turning the world into a huge hospital ward; almost all of life, from birth to death, has been turned into problems that medical professionals are expected to treat. Sick roles are forced on people. In effect, people have turned over their lives to what Illich calls the "biofascists."

Of the main evil results that Illich detects, I agree with his perception of the cultural effects of overreliance on medical professionals as a symptom of the dependency of man in an industrialized society. People are encouraged to become consumers of cures rather than advocates of changing morbid social political conditions.[12] Perhaps the height of this problem from a social point of view is the use of medicine by political systems to defeat any objection to a system, as is done in Russia. There objectors are classified as being mentally ill, and are drugged until their objections and sense of self fade into oblivion. Solzhenitsyn's accounts, the Nazi experiments, the use of medicine by rightist regimes in South America, and our own experiments on prisoners and children lend real credence to the danger of social control over medicine, as well as the overmedicalization of society. Recall that political objectors in the 1960s in this country were labeled by Vice-President Agnew as "sick".

Illich might gain more adherents to his view from medical practitioners if he also pointed out the deleterious effects of over medicalization on medicine itself. I have already indicated some of these. The point, though, is that increased dependency upon any one resource reduces flexibility and the chance for survival. If human beings feel less self-reliant because they depend on medical cures for everything that ails them, their self-determination flags. Overreacting, they view medicine as a commodity and treat it as an industrial product. Gene H. Stollerman, speaking in his capacity as president of the Society for Clinical Research, has said: "The emergence of a special advocacy for our patients as 'consumers' and the characterization of our activity as 'a product' are in themselves uncomfortable reminders of the increasingly industrial nature of medical practice."[13]

While Dr. Stollerman has harsh words for this conception of the medical profession, he does not spell out the major danger of viewing medicine as a commodity—namely, the loss of professional flexibility, to which I have already alluded. Another way of viewing the same danger is to consider how professional altruism, the desire to serve another without attention to one's own needs, diminishes in a consumer-product model of health care. Economic factors, rules about the buyer being wary of the product, enter the health care professional-patient relationship and destroy the trust necessary for good health. Competition, rather than compassion, results. So now doctors are being encouraged to countersue their patients. Professional resourcefulness, formerly stimulated by a compassionate altruism, is reduced, truncated, destroyed by the consumer-product model. Compassion is replaced by the threat of torts.

Finally, overmedicalization of society produces impossible pressures upon the health professions. Marx Wartofsky, among others, propounds the view that health and disease are social concepts. Hence, health care professionals are responsible for curing social ills. No matter how much attention is paid in the few years of medical training to social factors of disease and health, health professionals are singularly deficient in tools for curing social ills. But if we substitute for our former gods the man or woman in the white coat, we do indeed expect them to cure all our ills. Health professionals are not entirely faultless in creating this view of their profession, and are only now reaping the grim benefits of a modern American mythology.

THE GOALS OF MEDICINE AND SOCIETY

Any discussion of the goals of medicine and society will involve complex interactions because they both deal with fundamental needs and aspirations of man. Like the DNA molecule, the medicine-society molecule genetically predetermines man's self-image. Do the goals of medicine and the goals of society interlock? Do these goals mesh? Or are they a destructive symbiosis of clashing goals? Innocent enough on the surface, these questions, as we have already seen, have enormous consequences for political, social, and cultural life.

My thesis is this: the stated goals of society are ideals realized only in part and infrequently. The stated goals of medicine are virtually nonexistent. Medicine suffers from an abundance of means and a poverty of ends.[14] The actual goals of medicine and society do interlock, but these realized goals frequently clash with what can be envisioned as a proper direction for human life.

What, then, are the professed goals of society? This is a difficult question to answer. I think that some consensus about professed goals can be gained by looking at two theories of what is wrong with our civilization today. One theory is that of Bertrand Russell, the famous English philosopher and mathematician. Russell's view was that our civilization lacks cultural wisdom about the right ends of a human life, a wisdom that he believed science in itself cannot provide. In other words, mankind lacks the moral strength to carry out the insights gleaned from the sciences into a common moral policy. In Russell's view, there exists both information overload and moral incapacity. The other theory is posed by Karl Popper, another

English philosopher of science. In Popper's view, mankind has a great deal of moral enthusiasm, but a lack of true understanding. His point seems to echo a statement of Justice Brandeis in 1928: "The greatest dangers to liberty lurk in insidious encroachment by men of zeal, well-meaning, but without understanding." Russell's view, then, is that man is too smart for his moral britches; Popper, on the other hand, holds that mankind is morally energetic, but is just plain stupid.

Behind both of these theories lies an important assumption: the goals of a society involve a correct understanding of the right ends of human life and a moral policy by which to carry out these ends. Among the values inherent in such moral policy, I suggest the following: it is good to be healthy; it is good to have friends or community support; and it is good to have economic resources in order to live a virtuous life. Think for a moment about the enormous energy and human resources that go into achieving these values of health, community, and virtue. My own view is that we lack a proper understanding of how these values interlock, and we lack the mechanisms of an international moral policy to provide for these goods.

If the professed goal of human society is to recognize, enact, and reinforce the right ends of human life, what then are the real goals? After considerable thought, I tend to lean toward one answer: narcissism. In return for relinquishing part of our freedom to technologized and mechanized institutions, we receive the value of self-love, or self-pampering. If our dull jobs cause us even more dulling headaches, we can have instant pain-killing cures. If our breasts or scrota sag with age, we can have cosmetic surgery. If our sexual activity leads to irresponsibility, we can have the fetus removed from the scene. If our self-indulgence in food while others starve gives us gas, we have antacid tablets; if it produces obesity, we have drugs and surgery to cure that. If our work and marriage are boring, we can switch. If the television program gets too serious, we can switch the channel in favor of the more insipid Johnny Carson. If we do not like our house, our neighborhood, our country, we can dump them and move. If, in the end, we do not like ourselves, we can clothe, manicure, perfume, and truss ourselves into respectibility. Without belaboring the point, I suggest a clear trend in the goal of our society toward self-interest. The business world is always on top of these matters, and a recent market research study shows that products which increase pampering and self-indulgence are the best investments for the future.

But what are the professed goals of medicine? This question is doubly difficult. Not only does medicine suffer from a poverty of ends, but it also is not a monolithic discipline. Medicine embraces everything from public health sewage treatment to neurosurgery, from physical therapy to cancer treatment, from medical technicians to family practice. What is more, if the general notion of health is the goal of medicine, then few agree on its definition. It has become much easier to define specific diseases than health, even specific healths. In 1965 Clifton K. Meador, M.D., of the University of Alabama Medical Center, made a valiant effort toward defining nondisease entities, but his ideas have not caught on.[15]

To be sure, the professed goals of medicine are unclear. Eric Cassell is among the many physicians who try to articulate the goals of medicine from the standpoint of health and disease. In an early work, Cassell argues that the goal of medicine is healing, not necessarily curing. Illness, in this view, is the general feeling a patient has about the self, while a disease is a scientific name given to a specific malfunction of an organ or organ system. The goal of medicine would then be to cure the disease, if possible, but also to effect changes in the larger feeling of illness. As Cassell puts it, the latter action of medicine becomes an "applied moral philosophy":

> Medicine is inherently a moral profession: its practitioners are committed to action in the service of the good. Physicians assemble facts about the body and disease, and, on the basis of that technical knowledge, take action for the welfare and good of their patients. In short, we use technical means to achieve moral ends.[16]

Remarkably similar to the goals of society (namely, the formulation and encouragement of moral policy for the good of man), the ideal goals of medicine include a respect for living beings, good care, compassion, providing a measure of hope, seeking cure, and healing the whole person. The altruism of the profession is expressed, for example, in the Declaration of Geneva, often used in place of the Hippocratic Oath: "The health of my patient will be my first consideration. . . . Even under threat I will not use my medical knowledge contrary to the laws of humanity."

In a more recent publication, Cassell argues that the professed goal of medicine is actually autonomy.[17] Autonomy involves, as Dworkin suggests, both authenticity and freedom.[18] Illness has a negative impact on both.[19] Cassell claims that the physician can preserve autonomy by preserving the authentic personhood behind the illness and restoring independence by: (1) offering reasons for the disease; (2) acting on behalf of the damaged independent person; and (3) enhancing that person's ability to reason about goods.[20] In this line of argument, preserving life, prolonging life, and curing are subservient to the healing (autonomous preservation) task. Pellegrino and I also argue that the end of medicine is to heal the body, the self, and the social side of a person by working in and through the body.[21] This requirement gives specificity to medical acts. If one were to take Cassell's version at face value, the aim of medicine would not differ significantly from the aim of teaching or jurisprudence, or for that matter, child rearing.

If one accepts this line of argument, then, the goals of medicine and society on the level of what ought to occur are certainly congruent. Society should support and encourage autonomy. Medicine, by working toward healing, can support that autonomy and even restore it through its efforts on behalf of the body, the mind, and the person in social context. In face of this appealing idealism, one might echo Robert Louis Stevenson's words about physicians:

> There are men and classes of men that stand above the common herd: the soldier, the sailor, and the shepherd not infrequently; the artist rarely, rarelier still, the clergyman; the physician almost as a rule. . . . Generosity he has, such as is possible to those who practice an art, never to those who drive a trade; discretion, tested by a hundred secrets; tacts, tried in a thousand embarrassments and what are more important, Heraclean cheerfulness and courage.

But now the reality curtain must come down on these strawberry dreams. While it might be true that individual practitioners of medicine are often truly concerned about others, are humble and generous, cheerful and courageous, the profession is also filled with those who are greedy, self-centered, paternalistic, tactless, and ultimately concerned only with self-advancement and the curing of individual organ systems.

What is more, even those individuals within the profession who manage to maintain their altruism beyond formal training find it extremely difficult, often unbearable, to practice altruistic medicine in and among their peers, our medical institutions, and degree-granting agencies. On top of that, little reinforcement comes from patients who know that doctors rank among the highest paid professionals in the country, while adequate health care for all remains a politically embarrassing unfulfilled goal.

The myth of excellence about modern medicine should be questioned by the facts. Despite our economic outlays and advanced equipment, the truth is that our health care is in a state of crisis. Consider the view of Halsted R. Holman, M.D., professor of Medicine at Stanford, who writes:

> For years, as medical care expenditures have risen beyond the rate of inflation, there has been no direct relationship between expense and outcome. Longevity has changed little, and the major illnesses such as malignancy and cardiovascular disease remain unimpeded. Heralded preventive measures such as a multiphasic screening and modification of risk factors for cardiovascular disease yield limited benefit. Illness disproportionately affects the poor, major environmental and occupational causes of illnesses receive little attention and less action, and malpractice charges intensify. Clearly, there is a crisis in health care, both in its effect upon health and in its cost.[22]

Because it is so easy to add prophetic voice upon prophetic voice, I want simply to note how infrequently the real goals of medicine approach the professed ones. The times when the whole person is treated are rare; rarer still are the times when physicians even ask patients if they have any questions (a survey five years old showed only about ten percent of the time are patients asked.)[23] Sometimes, cases even occur like the one in Alabama when Dr. Bobby Merkle removed stitches from a boy's hand because of lack of payment.[24] Medicine, seen in this less attractive light, is in danger of coalescing with the real goals of society. In fact, it has already contributed to them as the examples I gave already show. I suggest that narcissism has little to do with the meaning of life and certainly little to do with the altruism necessary for the practice of the applied moral discipline of medicine.

What can be done? First, I think a closer examination of the goals of medicine and society is necessary; second, in line with

Cassell's thinking, medicine must clarify the meaning of health. In this way, it can avoid being pressured into responsibility for curing all the ills of society. Simultaneously, it will acquire a measure by which it can identify its real achievements and its real problems. If medicine could adopt the Aristotelean view that the job as a profession is not to make man healthy, but to put that man as far as may be possible on the road to health, then the process of healing could be viewed as simply that, a process involving the rich resources of modern medicine, the whole person of its practitioners, and the whole personality of those to be healed.

Because medicine maintains its responsibility to human need, it maintains an inherent conscience. Unlike the pure sciences, it can never depart from the human condition, even in its research activities. While the universalism of physics, for example, rests upon its humbling experience of not being able to relate its discoveries to something more profound (here I borrow from Rabi as quoted in *The New Yorker*, October 21, 1975, p. 94), medicine as a discipline acquires its universalism from the human condition. Its activity directly relates to one of the goals of human society and to the aspirations of mankind. For this reason, I am considerably more hopeful that medicine can overcome its present crisis than Illich might be.

APPROPRIATE GOALS OF SOCIETY AND MEDICINE

What ought to be the goals of technological society? Given the extent to which individual freedoms are curtailed by dependency on technological systems (even while choices of products may increase), it is tempting to think that autonomy ought to be the goal of society. But autonomy, however much we may value it, is deficient as an aim of society on at least two counts. First, autonomy is often loosely identified with personal or individual freedom. It rarely, if ever, is applied to groups or communities. But the goal of society ought to embrace both individuals and communities. Second, autonomy is often equated with the dignity of a person. Yet persons are more than autonomous entities. They are also under obligations to others both by contract and by nature; they are often motivated by needs, wants, and wishes that call forth the many and complex relations of dependency necessary for survival and fulfillment of the proper ends of a good human life. It is best, thus, to consider the goals of a technological society in the broadest terms possible and to concentrate one's energies on identifying specific ends of a good human life. The goal might, therefore, be as follows: to preserve those values that best support individual freedom and social adhesion.

Among such values is health, a value that is unimpeachably central to the well-being of individuals and groups. For this reason it is also the primary identifier for the appropriate goal for medicine. Medicine's goal is to heal. Because health is a foundational value for persons and groups, it is normally regarded by us (as evidenced in behavioral studies of attitudes) as a means for other more highly regarded values, such as freedom, mobility, strong family ties, and so on. Philosophers from Aristotle to Dewey have recognized this foundational status of health. It is a necessary, but not sufficient, condition for personal and social well-being. As behavioral studies also indicate, however, the foundational status of health in no way indicates secondary status when persons become ill. Almost universally in illness, health is ranked as a première value. One is willing to sacrifice personal freedoms and social ties in order to regain it, as happens when a patient enters a hospital. To reestablish health one must suffer *(pati),* become a patient. To become a patient is to become dependent on the expertise of others in a way one was formerly not.

Some moral anomalies are embodied in the idea of health or healing as the goal of medicine. First, health is an absolute value of the body. That is, the body chooses or selects health instinctively before there are any personal interpretations or assaults on it. Tissues regenerate. Antibodies are produced.[25] Second, and as consequence, the value of health is normative for persons and for medicine. By normative I mean that certain patterns of action are mandated by the value of health, among which are seeking help, offering assistance to those in pain, and so on. A second meaning of normative is also generated in the scientific classification of disease. The taxonomy of a person's disease created in the diagnostic process is such that the expert, the informed layperson, and often the patient can judge what is normal and what is abnormal.[26] Third, health is a moral value because it is beneficial for persons, for society, and for patients. Health is not only a biological condition, but as the aim of medicine and of the patients who enter the healing relationship, it is also morally beneficial.[27] Making the right and good decision for patients is, therefore, the act of medicine that stems from its end. Medicine is not morally neutral, but a good operative habit or, in Aristotelian terms, a virtue.[28] Fourth, as a consequence of the normative nature of health (in both senses) and its moral character, persons entering the medical relationship are subject to dependency on an expert, which has moral implications, two of which are that the relationship itself is governed by moral norms established by the goal of health and that the relationship must be temporary and/or adjustable. Ideally, health is restored, and the patient regains function and autonomy, as in the scenario I previously cited by Cassell. It is this ideal of temporariness that is shattered, of course, in the case of Grimes Posnovich that opened this essay.

Because health is simultaneously normative for the medical relationship and subject to personal and social interpretation, expert assumptions about the goal of medicine and patient assumptions clash. These clashes are most often the result of differing, nonexplicit conceptions of health. Since the goal of medicine is to restore health, this task must rest on dialogue to establish the parameters and functions both doctor and patient will assume to reach the goal. In some cases the patient rejects the primary value of health in favor of other values. Examples are the Jehovah's Witness who rejects life-saving blood transfusions, the aging patient who requests that he die in peace without being connected to machinery. In the main this rejection of health as a basic value usually occurs when the temporary, restorative mode of healing becomes a more permanent dependency on medical care.

Yet another moral problem occurs within the medical relationship itself. Because the patient is an impaired person and because correction of this impairment requires dependency on experts, an obligation to restore independence is imposed on the expert. With Pellegrino, I have called this the vulnerability axiom.[29] What is important is that this axiom arises from the value of health and the medical relationship, and a code of professional obligations can be developed from it rather than from canons of legal and economic concerns.

It is also important, and a matter of some debate, to recognize that health is not a totally relative or vacuous concept.[30]

On the one hand, the organic definienda of health can function as signposts for the dialogical negotiation between doctor and patient about the moral weight to be given health in comparison with other values (making the right and good decision for patients). On the other hand, these same biological definienda and the negotiated hermeneutic of health lend content to the World Health Organization definition of "complete physical, mental, and social well-being and not merely the absence of disease or infirmity."[31]

Health is a condition of well-being, a necessary condition and an absolute value. But it is not a sufficient condition. For this reason, in this essay I have proposed restoring health as the proper end of medicine and have explored its relation to the goals of society. I have tried to avoid the following three errors in this regard:

(1) The Error of Vacuity: To claim that the aim of medicine is to restore well-being or to restore autonomy is to ask more of the discipline and its agents than it or they can provide. These are more properly the aim of society itself.

(2) The Error of Social Relativism: To claim, as many contemporary philosophers of science do, that the aim of medicine is primarily social,[32] is to neglect the organic basis of disease and the corporeal identity of persons. Medicine must work in and through the body. While the scientific and axiological concepts of health and disease do function as an absolute ground for the proposed aim of medicine, health as a moral aim includes its negotiated interpretation occurring in the doctor-patient relation. In other words, health is absolute as a value to the body and to scientific medicine, but is simultaneously relative to the patient, the practitioner, and society because they can and do interpret its moral meaning for the person or group and determine its relative rank among other moral goods and values in the construction of a treatment plan. Thus, Grimes's longevity goal should have been balanced against at least some limited autonomy that he required as a person. He was, in my *Gedankexperiment,* willing to forgo some but not all freedoms in order to gain longevity.

(3) The Error of Neutrality: Moral neutrality, whatever its supposed merits when applied to the sciences, cannot be applied to medicine. Because of the normative nature of health, the necessity of negotiating both the meaning and the relative ranking of health-as-value in each individual instance, and be-

cause the vulnerability axiom is but one of a number of ethical middle principles that govern the medical transaction,[33] all actions of medicine as defined (making right and good decisions for patients) are moral—that is, involve values. As such these actions are subject to ethical analyses based not only on principles in various ethical systems, but also on axioms forged out of the warp and woof of the medical enterprise.

In this way the proposal of restoring health as the appropriate goal of medicine at once requires a moral analysis of the medical enterprise, an existential understanding of personal impairment and the relation of this impairment to other values, and an ordering of action according to these rational analyses. Medicine, like many other modern technological disciplines so construed and so dedicated, can offer us a list of the proper ends of a good human life from the agonies and triumphs of death and healing. But it should never be allowed to determine these ends. As David Lygre writes in his *Life Manipulation*, "Our tools for manipulating life need not rob us of our souls. In fact it is our ethical, social, and spiritual values—not our physical tools—that must command our future."[34]

NOTES

1. Examples are Ronald Rosenbaum and Susan Edmiston, "Dead Ringers," *Esquire* 85 (1976): 98–103; Patrick M. McGrady, Jr., "The American Cancer Society Means Well, but the Janker Clinic Means Better," *Esquire* 85 (1976): 111–14; Alexander Theroux, "The Shrink," *Esquire* 84 (1975): 166.

2. Nora Ephron, "The Mink Coat," *Esquire* 84 (1975): 118–20; John Sack, "Congratulations, Mr, and Mrs. Sack. You've Just Given Birth to an Eight-Pound, Eight-Ounce Slave," *Esquire* 85 (1976): 98–100, 112–21. Also cf. Urie Bronfenbrenner, *Two Worlds of Childhood: USSR and USA* (New York: Russell Sage Foundation, 1970).

3. As quoted in C. Schneiker, "An Abridged Collection of Interdisciplinary Laws," *The CoEvolution Quarterly* (Winter 1975): 138.

4. Don DeLillo, "Showdown at Great Hole," *Esquire* 85 (1976): 108–10; 134–38.

5. P. Siemer, "Now, About the Tricentennial," *Memphis Commercial Appeal*, July 5, 1976, p.4: "In the field of medicine, experts see the future as an era of increased lifespan, with Americans living routinely into their 100s; living tissue replacements, so much so that one prominent physician sees a black market in organs as 'inevitable'; artificial organs; breakthrough in genetics and aging, and the prevention or cure of some dread diseases. 'The human . . . will have infinite ways to devise techniques to avoid its demise and to encourage its survival,' said Dr. David Kipnis, Chairman of Washington University's Department of Internal Medicine. In the spirit of 'Future Shock,' Dr. Kipnis wonders if 21st Century physicians will deal with a whole host of 'coping' illnesses brought on by a more complicated society and simple survival in an increasingly regulated world."

6. Dennis Carlson, a physician on the faculty of Johns Hopkins University School of Medicine, has worked on the ways in which art and drama, including dance and music, have an impact on health. His findings clearly demonstrate the importance of viewing medicine's goal as aimed at the whole person, however that may be defined, and not just at a biological entity. See "Health, Art, and Drama: Underutilized Resources for Improved Quality of Life" in this volume, pp. 145–57.

7. R. Greene, M.D., writing in *Hospital Physician* (March 1976): 38, bemoans the loss of true clinical teaching in medical schools.

8. H. J. Geiger, M.D., professor of community medicine, in an article for the *N.Y. Times Book Review* on Ivan Illich's *Medical Nemesis* noted the impact of medicine on personal freedom. In the many reviews and diatribes caused by Illich's book, no one questioned the fundamental premise, that medicine's goals are intertwined with those of society and vice versa.

9. See Norman Birnbaum, "The Future of the Humanities," *Change* 7 (Summer 1975): 11–13, who explored the effect of fragmentation on the humanities and higher education. Nothing since that date, except perhaps for the movements relating philosophy to medicine and the humanities to the professions, has been written to invalidate his observations.

10. Although concern about malpractice seemed to reach an apogee in 1975 and 1976, the worry is still present today. Among the theories about why this concern appeared so volatile was that of Dr. M. Parrott, president of the American Medical Association in 1976, who thought malpractice resulted from the lack of appreciation for scientific method on the part of lawyers. Lawyers often claim that insurance companies are at fault. Neither of these theories is correct. The real reason for malpractice is that doctors and patients no longer share common values. Patients may expect too much from medicine, which in turn treats them as objects. Physicians do battle daily with the romantic visions of the gentle and kind physician who made housecalls every day (but who could not cure). This picture, common among patients and physicians, of a rosier and (therefore, they think) happier time, distorts the values patients and physicians actually bring to the relationship in this modern, technological society.

11. Robert P. Hudson, M.D., "How Real is Our Reverence for Life?" *Prism* (June 1975): 19–21; 58–59.

12. See reaction to Illich's talk at SUNY at Stony Brook after publishing *Medical Nemesis*. A report reached Memphis, Tennessee, in *Common Sense* (May 23, 1976, p. 8), entitled "Illich Attacks Medical Profession."

13. Gene H. Stollerman, "Consumerism and Clinical Investigation," *Journal of Laboratory and Clinical Medicine* 87 (1976): 179.

14. Edmund D. Pellegrino and David C. Thomasma, *A Philosophical Basis of Medical Practice* (New York: Oxford University Press, 1981).

15. Clifton K. Meador, "The Art and Science of Nondisease," *New England Journal of Medicine* 272 (1965): 92–95.

16. Eric J. Cassell, "Healing," *Hospital Physician* 4(1976): 28; also see his "Illness and Disease," *Hastings Center Report* 6 (1976): 27–37; *The Healer's Art* (New York: Lippincott, 1976). Robert P. Hudson provides a convenient sketch on the dilemmas of young medical students regarding health and disease. See "The Concepts of Disease," *Annals of Internal Medicine* 56(1966): 595–601.

17. Eric J. Cassell, "What is the Function of Medicine?" in *Death and Decision*, ed. E. McMullin (Boulder, Col.: Westview Press, 1978), pp. 35–44.

18. Gerald Dworkin, "Autonomy and Behavior Control," *Hastings Center Report* 6(1976): 23–28.

19. Cassell, *The Healer's Art*, pp. 47–83. This section covers the point that the sick are different from the well with respect to autonomy.

20. Cassell, "What is the Function of Medicine?" p. 42.

21. Pellegrino and Thomasma, *A Philosophical Basis.*

22. Halsted R. Holman, "The 'Excellence' Deception in Medicine," *Hospital Practice* 11 (April 1976): 11.

23. As reported in "Blame Misplaced in Pill Regimen," *Memphis Commercial Appeal,* May 30, 1976, p. 4.

24. Vanderbilt Hospital once threatened to stop treatment of a six-year-old boy because he could not pay for his cancer treatment. See *Memphis Commercial Appeal,* May 30, 1976. Incidents like these seem to have diminished in recent years.

25. Pellegrino and Thomasma, *A Philosophical Basis,* chap. 5.

26. Georges Canguilhem, *On the Normal and the Pathological* (Dordrecht, Holland: D. Reidel Publishing Co., 1978); H. Tristram Engelhardt, Jr., "The Concepts of Health and Disease," and M. W. Wartofsky, "Organs, Organisms and Disease: Human Ontology and Medical Practice," in *Evaluation and Explanation in the Biomedical Sciences,* ed.H. Tristram Engelhardt, Jr., and Stuart F. Spicker (Boston/Dordrecht: D. Reidel Publishing Co., 1975), pp. 125–42 and pp. 67–84, respectively.

27. Pellegrino and Thomasma, *A Philosophical Basis,* chap. 8.

28. Edmund D. Pellegrino, "The Anatomy of Clinical Judgments: Some Notes on Right Reason and Right Action," in *Clinical Judgment: A Critical Appraisal,* ed. H. T. Engelhardt, Jr., Stuart F. Spicker, and Bertrand Towers (Boston/Dordrecht: D. Reidel Publishing Co., 1979), pp. 169–94.

29. David Thomasma and Edmund D. Pellegrino, "Philosophy of Medicine as Source for Medical Ethics," *Metamedicine* 2(1981): 5–11; Pellegrino and Thomasma, *A Philosophical Basis,* chap. 8.

30. See the critical responses to our *Metamedicine* paper cited in note 29 by Moskop, McCollough, Wear, and Whitebeck in the same issue, as well as our "Response to Our Commentators" in that issue.

31. "Preamble to the Constitution of the World Health Organization," *The First Ten Years of the World Health Organization* (Geneva: WHO, 1958), p. 459.

32. Principal among these is Alasdair MacIntyre, "Medicine Aimed at the Care of Persons Rather Than What. . . ?" delivered at the Conference on Changing Values in Medicine, Cornell University, New York City, November 13, 1979. See also the response by E. D. Pellegrino, "Treating the Patient as Person: Philosophical Groundings," from the same conference. These papers will be published by the University of Chicago Press.

33. David Thomasma, "The Possibility of a Normative Medical Ethics," *Journal of Medicine and Philosophy* 5 (1980): 249–59.

34. David Lygre, *Life Manipulation* (New York: Walker and Co., 1979), p. 5.

The Phenomenon of Medicine: Of Hoaxes and Humor

RICHARD M. ZANER

School of Medicine, Vanderbilt University

In 1492, serious efforts were made to save the failing life of Pope Innocent VIII. With the patient in a deep coma and a deathly, bloodless pallor over his body, the effort to revive him took the form of pouring down his throat the blood of three healthy young men. It was no use, of course; he immediately died, as did the three donors. The moral of the tale for the present effort: even though circumstances may at times seem to call for desperate measures, one should be wary of conventional diagnoses and remedies. In the present case, the phenomenon—medicine—is unmanageably complex. Not unlike the goodly Pope, medicine is said to be suffering critically, in spite of otherwise robust signs of health.[1] Rather than trying drastic measures, then, and possibly risking more than what was initially bargained for, it seems wiser to invest in a different effort: a sort of phenomenological etiology. What follows, at least, is the sketch of such a trial.

For all its evident complexities, modern medicine presents certain prominences. One of these is quite remarkable: medicine and its underpinning, basic health sciences, seem intractably set in a version of Cartesian dualism.[2] Edmund Pellegrino's observation is appropriate: medicine today is "a fusion of the neo-Hippocratic spirit with a new, matured Cartesian conviction that human illness can be described in physicochemical and quantified terms."[3] Thus Macfarlane Burnet states without hesitation that

> Medicine in general has changed its whole pattern since in the last

> fifty years infection, physical injury, and malnutrition have become matters to be prevented or treated on a sound scientific basis, and effectively. What remains to be dealt with clinically is almost wholly dependent on the genetic constitution of the individual and his or her response to the social environment. . . . We have to face, more critically than it has yet been looked at, the likelihood that human behavior is predominantly, and in critical matters wholly, determined at the genetic level. Here, if anywhere, a modern philosopher will be most likely to find his approach to the problem of evil in the world. We may find in the end that war and evil, pain and disease, aging and death were inevitable as soon as a working pattern of life with DNA, ATP, and protein as enzyme had been devised.[4]

Or, in the words of Wilder Penfield,

> Because it seems to me certain that it will always be quite impossible to explain the mind on the basis of the neuronal action within the brain, and because it seems to me that the mind develops and matures independently throughout an individual's life as though it were a continuing element, and because a computer (which the brain is) must be programmed and operated by an agency capable of independent understanding, I am forced to choose the proposition that our being is to be explained on the basis of two fundamental elements.[5]

The physician is called on to become an adept clinical observer, and at the same time to interpret his findings in physicochemical and quantified terms. While the practice of medicine is often accomplished with great sensitivity and insight, it seems that such clinical descriptions only rarely find their way into the theory of medicine.[6]

The relatively recent prominence of psychiatry in medicine, even if it be a spectral rather than an actual force, may function as a corrective to reductivistic-materialistic ontology.[7] There can be no reckoning with medicine without taking into account its prevailing tendency to interpret human affliction this way. Thus, medicine presents us with an established view of the human body, the human psyche, and of their relationships. This view has been constructed historically and presents distinctive problems that would not arise from another view of illness or impairment. It understands the human body as a strictly biological affair, innocent of values, personal or social, and to be explained as far as possible without reference to persons, souls, psyches, spirits, minds, or even social life.[8] These aspects of life are not proper subjects for physical or medical science. Indeed, so far as psychic disturbances are medically treatable, their treatment and explanation are to be taken as having biological or chemical causes. To the extent that afflictions do not seem amenable to such a model, one confronts a main tension in medicine, the dilemma of not knowing how to proceed. However clinical practice presents this tension, medicine focuses on the various systems, organs, structures, and functions of the body. It is thus necessary to ask, What is the use of the human body for medicine's explanatory interest?

Indirection will help to elicit the phenomenon. Paul Ramsey has made the following observation in another connection:

> In the second year anatomy course, medical students clothe with "gallows humor" their encounter with the cadaver which once was a human being alive. That defense is not to be despised; nor does it necessarily indicate socialization in shallowness. . . . Even when dealing with the remains of the long since dead, there is special tension involved . . . when performing investigatory medical actions involving the face, the hands, and the genitalia. This thing-in-the-world that was once a man alive we still encounter as once a communicating being, not quite as an object of research or instruction. Face and hands, yes; but why the genitalia? Those reactions must seem incongruous to a resolutely biologizing age. For a beginning of an explanation, one might take up the expression "carnal knowledge" . . . and behind that go to the expression *"carnal conversation,"* an old legal term for adultery, and back of both to the Biblical word "know." . . . Here we have an entire anthropology impacted in a word, not a squeamish euphemism. In short, in those reactions of medical students can be discerned a sensed relic of the human being bodily experiencing and communicating, and the body itself uniquely speaking.[9]

Wishing to evoke the "felt difference between life and death," Ramsey emphasizes that this difference makes itself known even in the case of the cadaver. To be sure, the incommensurable contrast between life and death is met most dramatically with the "newly dead": if the cadaver produces gallows humor, the mangled body lying on the ER stretcher awakens dread and awe. Both, however, suggest an almost haunting presence of once-living flesh—of body gestures, attitudes, glances, movements—that a "resolutely biologizing age" may too easily, too readily ignore or suppress.

Although Ramsey's own view of the "body itself uniquely speaking" reasserts the very dualism he otherwise seeks to dispel,[10] this "gallows humor" suggests not only "an entire anthropology"—the implications of which seem to me to differ from what Ramsey has in mind—but also indicates that the cadaver is indeed an "object of research and instruction." Of course, medical students should learn from dissections, just as investigators learn from research on such cadavers. But the obviousness of this reasoning should give us pause. How does it happen that the live human body can be explained by the dead human body?[11]

While it may seem an exaggeration to suggest that the dead body functions as the model for the live human body—the corpse for the soma—it is equally distorting to dismiss the theory out of hand. Although a "special tension" exists when performing investigatory medical actions on the face, hands, and genitalia, it is by such actions that the body seems to become finally intelligible to us. In contrast, Hans Jonas writes that in classical times

> . . . it was the corpse, this primal exhibition of "dead" matter, which was the limit of all understanding and therefore the first thing not to be accepted at its face-value. Today the living, feeling, striving organism has taken over this role and is being unmasked as a *ludibrium materiae,* a subtle hoax of matter. Only when a corpse is the body plainly intelligible: then it returns from its puzzling and unorthodox behavior of aliveness to the unambiguous, "familiar" state of a body within the world of bodies, whose general laws provide the canon of all comprehensibility. To approximate the laws of the organic body to this canon, i.e., to efface in *this* sense the boundaries between life and death, is the direction of modern thought on life as a physical fact. Our thinking today is under the ontological dominance of death. . . . All modern theories of life are to be understood against this backdrop of an ontology of death, from which each single life must coax or bully its lease, only to be swallowed up by it in the end.[12]

Thus, Jonas emphasizes that life constitutes the major theme and most pressing issue of modern times. As I see it, though, Jonas does not suggest that death, and much less dying, are thereby comprehended. Rather, the deadness of a cadaver is equivalent to the now "familiar" state of a body within a world of bodies. It is a piece of physical matter. Hence, the shock and stark enigma of death in our times is quite as much a *ludibrium materiae* as is life: matter is neither deanimate nor exanimate; it neither feels nor desires nor strives, neither lives nor dies. What is additionally intriguing about Jonas's point is the irony in his equivocation on death: the deadness of material particles and the death exhibited by the human corpse. The one is not the other, nor does dead matter as such evoke humor, much less gallows humor.

The equivocation, however, is suggestive in several unexpected ways. Modern medicine has increasingly become a crisis-centered discipline, evident not only from stereotyped portrayals in the media but equally from the emphasis in our medical schools. Its central focus (expressed, for example, by modes and quantity of funding, by the stress on clinical encounters, as also by the continuing and considerable pressures for developments of still more potent technologies and medical regimens) is disease, illness, injury, or affliction. Despite the fact that the bulk of the time most physicians spend with patients deals with mundane complaints and gripes, and very little on actual crises, medicine's principal public and encouraged image is of a discipline (a science, indeed) on the critical edge of life and death, warring constantly and valiantly against an aggressive, impersonal, and intractable enemy. Such images come quickly to mind and need not be repeated here. Suffice it to say that the humdrum, the prosaic, and the mundane have little place either in medical education or in much of the acquired self-understanding of health professionals. The prominence of combative, military, or warfare metaphors is clear enough, as are the various values they naturally evoke: bravery, perseverance, valor in the face of overwhelming and implacable odds.

My point is only that such metaphors are understandable the moment we recognize that they have their source in that subtle hoax of matter. Just as life, by Jonas's account, is puzzling and unorthodox, so must death be profoundly enigmatic—manageable, if you will, only when ultimately modeled as disease, something therefore to be, and indeed able to be, conquered like any other disease. In somewhat less dramatic and scientifically defensible terms, death becomes the unsurprising consequence of aging, or the result of "genetic errors in somatic cells."[13] "Death," Burnet claims, "is the culmination of maturity and old age, and I suspect that our reactions to the actualities of dying are determined by the genes we were born with to the same degree as any other aspect of our behavior."[14]

Thus has our own mortality become medicalized, rendered (so far as possible) familiar by being placed beside other enemies to be combatted.[15] For disease, like genetic error, seems able to be accommodated to materiality and is explainable finally by reduction to the same kind of "familiar" physical universe. But so too does life seem similarly accountable, and the metaphors come full circle (however viciously it may be). Thus life itself is a constant struggle for survival, ultimately against death, and medicine comes to be seen as serving the now-familiar and supposedly natural functions of evolution. Indeed, thanks to remarkable developments in genetics, it is increasingly commonplace to find it believed, as in the writing of Sir John Eccles, that

> planned genetic manipulation now replaces the natural process of biological mutation by chance. . . . [M]an has taken over control of the biological processes of differentiation, multiplication and survival. Biology is not completely frozen at the end of the evolutionary era. Rather it is now enslaved for man's purposes so that useful species are deliberately changed by genetic engineering in order that they can be more useful for exploitation.[16]

To witness the workings of such metaphors is to notice the fulfillment of Bacon's combative word usage: knowledge and power become one in the struggle to conquer man's otherwise endemically vulnerable and helpless condition. Medicine in its modern form, while it comprehends neither life nor death, yet has become one of the major forces for the understanding of the nature of body and mind, and thereby for altering human social and individual life. To the precise extent that its exercise of power (as Bacon already envisaged, Comte preached, and the twentieth century has begun to realize) is successful in combatting afflictions, as it surely has been in many ways, it has understandably accrued immense social prominence and prestige; medicine is, after all, one of the few (if not the sole) remaining sources of social authority in our culture.

We must not lose sight of several phenomena here. First, and in a way paramount, gallows humor and its underlying consort, the *ludibrium materiae,* mark out both life and death as enigmatic. A second phenomenon is medicine's accepted view of human reality, a view that is historical and constructed—an artifact. Third, historically medicine has become, especially during the last century, a human engagement of immense power and authority. In an age that has witnessed the flight of the gods, norms, and the elders, and that has seen the norms of transcendence and tradition steadily diminish and disperse, medicine—the discipline seemingly most directly attentive to life, death, affliction, guilt, failure—has come to assume the place of these basic conditions of human beings. But medicine, girded with the armor of biomedical science, is itself beset with endemic dilemmas, which themselves are historical phenomena. I want to take up these three phenomena, but in reverse order and only briefly.

H. Tristram Engelhardt, Jr., has pointed out that "medicine is the most revolutionary of human technologies. It does not sculpt statues or paint paintings: it restructures man and man's life. . . . In short, medicine is not merely a science, not merely a technology. . . . Medicine is the art of remaking man, not in the image of nature, but in his own image; medicine operates with an implicit idea of what man *should* be."[17]

Medical research has made it possible for the personal and social aspects of sexuality to be separated from its reproductive aspect. Consequently, human life has been decisively altered, with changes occurring in family structure, educational policy, child-rearing, and population planning. Even new issues have been generated, such as the rights of fetuses and the rights of certain persons to reproduce. Indeed, technological and biomedical prowess makes it currently plausible not only to conceive and practice genetic control of future humanity (to take our own evolution in hand),[18] not only to conceive and practice behavior control on individuals and even on entire populations (through psychopharmacological intervention, for example), but even also to conceive that our own mortality may be subject to medical control (taking death as a kind of disease or result of genetic error).[19]

Not only does such potential control force medicine itself to change,[20] but it also implies the power to alter, perhaps irrevocably and for better or worse, our very capacity to reckon with and to understand medicine—and thereby, our ability to know ourselves. This power has the capacity to cancel out all knowledge of having been used. It is, as Hans Jonas has argued, the drastically enhanced scale of technological intervention into nature, society, and the lives of individuals that forcibly reveals their critical vulnerability—a vulnerability "unsuspected before it began to show itself in damage already done."[21] Indeed, Jonas emphasizes what he terms the inherently "utopian" drift of our modern technological actions:

> . . . technological power has turned what used and ought to be tentative, perhaps enlightening, plays of speculative reason into competing blueprints for projects, and in choosing between them we have to choose between extremes of remote effects. . . . Living now constantly in the shadow of unwanted, built-in, automatic utopianism, we are constantly confronted with issues whose positive choice requires supreme wisdom—an impossible situation for man in general, because he does not possess that wisdom, and in particular for contemporary man, who denies the very existence of its object: viz., objective value and truth. We need wisdom most when we believe in it least.[22]

Medicine's focus is the human being, individually and socially, but especially, in our culture, it is on human afflictions and disruptions in personal and social life. Medicine's design, however, is not merely to treat; rather, it remakes and thereby is itself remade. That is, medicine and its focus are historical in specific ways. But that historicity did not emerge in the twentieth century, even though the impetus provided by biomedicine and its associated technology surely gave it unique prominence in our times. The historical-cultural texture that makes such an impetus possible in the first place was already at hand. As J. H. van den Berg has convincingly suggested in his remarkable conception of "metabletics,"[23] this may well be found in the historical division of the human context, whose beginnings occur at least 300 years before Descartes's metaphysical formalization of the schism.

If we would understand the dualism specific to modern times, van den Berg argues, we need to turn to medicine and especially to return to the beginnings of West European anatomy, when in 1306 Mundinus first cut into a human cadaver. His disciple, Vigevano, published an anatomical treatise in 1345 that included a number of illustrations. The first shows Vigevano next to an upright cadaver, which he has begun to open with a knife. As van den Berg explains:

> One would expect Vigevano to look at the knife. But he does not. He looks at the closed eyes of the dead man. He has a relationship with the corpse, with the man of that corpse, with this deceased fellow-human being. He puts his left hand in an affectionate, intimate manner around the dead man's body.[24]

Later, in 1543, Andreas Vesalius published a far more sophisticated text on anatomy. In one drawing Vesalius, the anatomist, looks out at the viewer while holding an arm cut open and displaying a number of details, as if inviting us to look at, to look into, the dissected arm. If one believes that the soul is in the body, the anatomist in effect is implying that all one finds when looking into the body is more body. No soul can be found. Here we face an anatomical preparation: the full corpse seems no longer of central interest either to Vesalius or, presumably, to the viewer. There is a thing, the arm, separated from the dead man. As van den Berg remarks, comparing the two drawings separated by 200 years, we see "that man has been alienated from his own body . . . that man has changed, has become two, has been divided into two parts: body and soul."[25]

Dating from and after this period, an elemental distress affecting the soul becomes evident. Scarcely a century after Descartes, this internal schism shows up explicitly and is for the first time formally termed *neurosis* by George Cheyne in his *The English Malady* (1733). Indeed, during Descartes's own time, William Harvey (1628) had declared not only that the human heart is a hollow muscle, but is a pump—hardly the seat of human faith, emotion, and feeling that it once had been considered. At the same time, several significant synchronic events sought to rescue, so it almost seems, the old-fashioned heart: Jean Eudes inaugurated the Order of the Sacred Heart, but Pascal also probed the logic of the heart. By the 1780s, Mesmer had discovered among some of his patients what he called a "magnetic sleep," resulting from what he thought was his magnetic power; Puységur (1784) discovered the same ability, calling it "spontaneous somnabulism." In 1786, Jean Paul Richter had talked about the *Doppelgänger,* and shortly afterward it was described by Ludwig Tieck (1791). By the end of the eighteenth century, the human soul had "turned into a double existence . . . split into two."[26]

In the next century, Kierkegaard wrote in his singular way about the despair affecting inwardness, and by the end of the nineteenth century, Freud's attention was drawn to the internal divisions of the psyche on which he put characteristic stress on the prevalence of the unconscious and its governance by that rudimentary neuter, the Id *(das Es)*. The human self effectively had become a fundamentally pathological entity. By the mid-1940s this psychic neuroticism became conceived, by Rogers and Sullivan, for instance, as an interpersonal, and no longer a merely intrapsychic, phenomenon. Normal human life had itself become pathological, and crisis had become normal.

Van den Berg argues that this history (which, he contends, is a history of anthropathology) is synchronously matched in other crucial cultural events: in painting, for instance, with the emancipation of the landscape; in theology, with the desacralization of the cosmos (within which one finds Eudes's and Pascal's appeals to the heart); in industrialization, whose first use of the flying shuttle came in the same year that Cheyne described the English malady (1733); and in still other respects. What we witness, in short, is

> a steadily growing separation of man and the universe. Synchronically there is an equally steady growth in the separation of mind and body. The human subject is being driven into a corner which is getting smaller and smaller and there, in that little corner, begins the pathology of the human subject. Then the old elements [earth, air, fire, water] are chased out of the universe, and when in this universe, which has been severed from man, the new elements appear, their atoms are split into tiny, the tiniest particles, and pathology threatens to overwhelm the subject. Today we know that our relations [with others] are ruled by the abnormal.[27]

These historical changes in human life cannot be understood merely as ephemeral variations on an underlying, unchanging human nature; rather, they are genuine, essential *emergents*.[28] Human life is thus historical. Indeed, so are the various understandings of human life historical; the very idea of "naturezing" human life (Husserl's "naturalization of consciousness") is itself an historical consequence of genuine changes in human reality. In these terms, too, the main focus of medicine on affliction and disease is the historical consequence of the same changes. As Husserl pointed out in 1910, the naturalization of consciousness depends strictly upon the discovery of nature in the modern sense—and, we should add, in the sense set out by the Cartesian dualism: nature as measurable extension, which was deepened lastingly in medicine, despite disagreements and uncertainties over the immaterial soul, in the century following Descartes.[29]

What Jonas calls the *ludibrium materiae,* and which I think must be extended to include death as well as life, may well begin to make its appearance, not with the Cartesian bifurcation nor with the emergence of physics and astronomy shortly before that time, but with the medical-anatomical intrusions into the human cadaver. For what begins to withdraw between the time of Mundinus and that of Vesalius is not only the vivid presence of the soul of the now-dead man; not only the lively appearance of the dead man's body; but also the vivid presence of the other person. With waning life, there fades as well the unique look and lift of a fellow man, and hence the mutuality of fellow-feeling. How it occurred that the physician-now-turned-anatomist would thereupon feel able and free to dissect the once-living and now-stilled flesh of the other—that is, how the *soma* becomes cadaver and thus available for dissection and anatomical presentation—I do not rightly know. But once it did occur, we note both the vestiges of fellow-feeling (with Mundinus's eyes still looking into the dead man's eyes) and the critical turning-away from the humanness of the body; which becomes now a mere cadaver (with Vesalius). That is, the subtle hoax of matter is most prominent precisely with this cadaver, this thing; it is this phenomenon that prepares the way to the later Cartesian conception of matter as mere extension (which is neither *de*animate nor *ex*animate, but *in*animate), not the reverse. Matter seems modeled less on atomistic doctrines and far more on what is now definitely a cadaver, vacant of life; yet it is that entity which still remains a relic of a once-alive and communicating person.

Even patients suffering from paresis in a limb undergo a marked attitude change toward the now-unfeeling limb, and, from this experience, we may learn a good deal about that subtle hoax. As Herbert Plügge notes, such a limb takes on an aspect of

> objective thinglikeness, such as an importunate heaviness, burden, weight, with the quality of a substance that feels [for the patient as for the physician] essentially strange, wooden, like plaster of paris,

in any event as largely space-filling and hence not altogether as a part of ourselves.[30]

It may well have been the nature talked about by the physician and anatomist that prepared the way for the nature of the physicist in modern times.

To be sure, there are numerous other events that went into this subtle and complex historical separation of mind and body; still, it seems clear that those first dissections are critical milestones (van den Berg) in this history. With the anatomical opening up of the body, furthermore, the fateful path for conceiving material nature as sheer, quantitative stuff in motion has been opened up as well. But at the same time, that elusive lift of the alive, embodied person, that insubstantial and fugitive soul, becomes ever more unsure:[31] a subterfuge of mere matter whose only home became, after being divided from its body and its world, that oddly uncompelling metaphysical substance, the *res cogitans,* which was striving to reach beyond itself to the world with clever argument and its own internal ideas but succeeding only by reliance on what then remained of transcendent benevolence. With the stripping away of the otherwise obvious opulence of animate life from nature, and the wealth of human experience as well relegated to the strictly subjective regions, there begins what van den Berg calls "the pathology of the human subject":

> . . . we would never be talking about mental health if we had not already for some hundred years been suffering from a general and in some ways gentle disease that encompasses our world. The first, most important symptom that there is something wrong with our *mental health* lies in the word "mental." Yes, if we are asked to live *mentally,* that is, as a *soul,* in a strange anatomical body, in a strange chemical-physical world, nobody can expect us to live in good health.[32]

The gallows humor so prominent in gross anatomy labs, just as the special tension subtly felt by researchers and instructors, thus assumes a deeper significance. The humor is, as it must be, profoundly reflexive. It is an ironic play whose set is the dissecting room and its carts; whose supporting cast, bedecked with tools and gowns, are the budding dissectors; and whose central characters and theme are the cadavers, only barely distinct from the carts that bear them. But in that bare difference is precisely the reflexive irony: as a relic of a man once alive, the corpse is a haunting presence to the anatomist of himself, a faint but telling reminder of intimacies now foreclosed and fellow-feelings now forbidden. That difference, however, has become an historically bare difference, the body a complex of systems and functions, and therewith the gallows humor. There is further irony in the young Vesalius stealthily stripping away part by part the body of a thief hanging on a gallows, in order to assemble his first full cadaver in his study.

To take medicine as a phenomenon is in part to be confronted by the significance of a certain conception about human life. Before criticizing that view—a critique, we must swiftly remind ourselves, that also has its sources in the very same history it critiques[33]—it seems to me imperative to clarify and explore it as an historical artifact.[34] I have here merely made a few suggestions, picking up on the most fruitful leads already advanced by others. I have also implied that this task falls squarely within the central thematics of Husserlian phenomenology. One might notice, however, how few Husserlian terms have found their way into this venture. For that, I offer neither consolation nor excuse, only a reminder of another side of my opening tale about the too-hasty ministrations of the Pope's attendants, who were too eager to suffuse their patient's body with living blood. Like them, we all at times are too quick to testify to the inadequacy and shortcomings of the old ways. After all, the attendants' idea was not altogether outrageous. The Pope was in dire need of new blood, but the attendants did not fully understand just how this could be accomplished, and it seems clear that refinements were needed. This is exactly what Husserlian phenomenology intrinsically demands of itself all the time: it keeps the phenomenon in question present at all times and attends most carefully the ways by which it is presented and the evidence for it.

Beyond this, it is the context of dealing corporeally with one another—in clinical medicine—that seems to me so significant for philosophy. Indeed, it is that type of skin trade that more than anything else exhibits the presence of philosophy for actual human life.

NOTES

1. Peter Schuck, "A Consumer's View of the Health Care System," *Ethics of Health Care* (Washington, D.C.: Institute of Medicine, National Academy of Sciences, 1974), pp. 95–118.

2. See John C. Eccles, *The Human Mystery* (Berlin: Springer-Verlag, 1979), and Wilder Penfield, *The Mystery of the Mind: A Critical Study of Consciousness and the Human Brain* (Princeton, N.J.: Princeton University Press, 1975).

3. Edmund Pellegrino, *Medicine and Philosophy: Some Notes on the Flirtations of Minerva and Aesculapius* (Philadelphia, Pa.: Society for Health and Human Values, 1974), p. 11.

4. Macfarlane Burnet, *Endurance of Life: The Implications of Genetics for Human Life* (London: Cambridge University Press, 1978), p. 2.

5. Wilder Penfield, *The Mystery of the Mind* (Princeton, N.J.: Princeton University Press, 1975), p. 80.

6. See Gerhard Bosch, *Infantile Autism: A Clinical and Phenomenological/Anthropological Investigation Taking Language as the Guide,* trans. D. and I. Jordan (Berlin: Springer-Verlag, 1970).

7. See Hans Jonas, *The Phenomenon of Life: Toward a Philosophical Biology* (New York: Harper and Row, 1966), and Leon Kass, "Regarding the End of Medicine and the Pursuit of Health," *The Public Interest* 40 (1975): 11–42.

8. See Andre Hellegers, "The Beginnings of Personhood: Radical Considerations," *The Perkins Journal* 27 (1973): 16–19.

9. Paul Ramsey, "The Indignity of 'Death with Dignity,'" *The Hastings Center Report* 4 (1974): 59.

10. See my *The Context of Self: A Phenomenological Inquiry Using Medicine as a Guide* (Athens: Ohio University Press, 1981), chap. 2.

11. See my "The Other Descartes and Medicine," in *Phenomenology and the Understanding of Human Destiny,* ed. Stephen Skousgaard (Washington, D.C.: University Press of America and the Center for Advanced Research in Phenomenology, 1981).

12. Jonas, *The Phenomenon of Life,* pp. 12, 15.

13. Burnet, *Endurance of Life,* p. 75.

14. Ibid., p. 88.

15. See Ivan Illich, *Medical Nemesis: The Expropriation of Health* (London: Calder and Boyars, 1975).

16. Eccles, *The Human Mystery,* p. 120; see also pp. 49–97.

17. H. Tristram Engelhardt, Jr., "The Philosophy of Medicine: A New Endeavor," *Texas Reports on Biology and Medicine* 31 (1973): 445.

18. Eccles, *The Human Mystery,* p. 120.

19. See Hans Jonas, *Philosophical Essays: From Ancient Creed to Technological Man* (Englewood Cliffs, N.J.: Prentice-Hall, 1974), pp. 12–18.

20. Engelhardt, "The Philosophy of Medicine," pp. 446–47.

21. Jonas, *Philosophical Essays,* p. 9.

22. Ibid., p. 18.

23. J. H. van den Berg, "A Metabletic-Philosophical Evaluation of Mental Health," in *Mental Health: Philosophical Perspectives,* ed. H. Tristram Engelhardt, Jr., and Stuart F. Spicker (Dordrecht, Holland: D. Reidel Publishing Co., 1978), pp. 121–35.

24. Ibid., p. 124.

25. Ibid., p. 127.

26. Ibid., p. 128.

27. Ibid., p. 134.

28. Ibid., p. 122.
29. See Lester S. King, *The Philosophy of Medicine, The Early Eighteenth Century* (Cambridge, Mass.: Harvard University Press, 1978).
30. "Man and His Body," in *The Philosophy of the Body*, ed. Stuart F. Spicker (Chicago: Quadrangle Books, 1970), p. 296.
31. See King, *Philosophy of Medicine*, pp. 15–41, 125–51.
32. "A Metabletic-Philosophical Evaluation," p. 135.
33. See my "Synchronism and Therapy," in *Mental Health: Philosophical Perspectives*, ed. H. Tristram Engelhardt, Jr. and Stuart F. Spicker (Dordrecht, Holland: D. Reidel Publishing Co., 1978), pp. 137–42.
34. See van den Berg, "A Metabletic-Philosophical Evaluation," p. 127.

Scientific Views of Human Nature: Implications for the Ethics of Technological Intervention

JAMES E. TROSKO

Michigan State University

> If we want to discover what man amounts to, we can only find it in what men are: and what men are, above all other things, is various. It is in understanding that variousness—its range, its nature, its basis, and its implications—that we shall come to construct a concept of human nature that has both substance and truth.
>
> C. Geertz, "The Impact of the Concept of Culture on the Concept of Man"

Society today is suffering both ecological and psychosocial crises because of the institutionalized intervention into human lives by powerful scientific and technological means. Phrases such as the "failure of nerve,"[1] "future shock,"[2] and "civilization malaise"[3] have been coined to convey the feeling that a psychic vacuum seems to have been created when experiences shaped by technological means and scientific knowledge no longer make sense to the individual. Seyyed Nasr eloquently describes this plight:

> The confrontation between man's own inventions and manipulations in the form of technology and human culture as well as the violent effect of the application of man's acquired knowledge of nature to the destruction of the natural environment have reached such proportions that many people in the modern world are at last beginning to question the validity of the conception of man held in the West since the rise of modern civilization. But to discuss such a

vast problem in a meaningful and constructive way, one cannot but begin by clearing the ground of the obstacles which he himself has kindled by allowing himself to forget who he is. Having sold his soul, in the manner of Faust, in order to gain dominion over the natural environment, he has created a situation in which the very control of the environment is turning into its strangulation, bringing in its wake not only ecocide but also ultimately suicide.[4]

My thesis is that the values which govern the use of that technology stem from erroneous views of human nature. Recycling pop bottles and training more psychiatrists will not solve our problems until we recognize that their root cause is our own view of our nature and our relationship to the physical and psychosocial environment. T. Colwell elaborates further on the cause of our contemporary problems:

. . . And it is rooted in a view of the man-Nature relationship which is dualistic in holding that the means of technological advance can be derived from Nature, but the ends which direct it cannot. Since the consequences of our technological means have produced the ecological crisis, it follows that the ends we have followed are suspect by implication. The search for a new theory of man's relationship to Nature, therefore, centers around the search for a new conception of the ends and values which guide the means we employ.[5]

In essence, the failure of social policies of human intervention such as law, health care delivery, penal correction, industrial or agricultural practices, and educational guidelines reflect political ideologies based on views of human nature that are not consistent with scientific evidence. Philip Rhinelander has pointed out the importance of the views of human nature:

Whitehead would have agreed, I think, that it is impossible to put forward any political or moral theories without making some assumptions about the nature of man. The concept or model may be awkward; it may be slippery; it may be indefinite. But since we cannot avoid employing some model of man, tacitly if not explicitly, it is important to be aware of what we are doing and to consider what implications may be latent in the models we have available for use.[6]

In *The Perfectibility of Man,* John Passmore has cited the influences of various views of nature from a Western, historical perspective. Bin-Ky Tan has shown how several conflicting views of human nature influenced the relationship of the individual human being to society in Eastern cultures.[7] Edmund Pellegrino has explained how various historical views of human nature have shaped concepts of health and disease, which, in turn, have molded quite diverse practices of medicine.[8] Recently, Albert Bandura has sought to examine the views of human nature conveyed by various psychological and behavioral theories.[9]

Since, as stated by James Drane, "every ethic is founded in a philosophy of man, and every philosophy of man points toward ethical behavior,"[10] we must try to integrate scientific knowledge bearing on human nature into a meaningful philosophy to germinate humane "moral" values. In light of contemporary events, such as the Vietnam War, the Watergate Affair, massive global pollution, overpopulation, and the energy crisis, the classical "well-springs" of moral values and behavior are conspicuously open to suspicion. That we are witnessing what might be referred to as "moral bankruptcy" is not surprising since we do not share a meaningful view of human nature. The absence of a clear view (as well as the existence of many conflicting views) will inevitably lead to moral chaos. If we are indeed serious about the amoral and immoral behavior of human beings that leads to the repression of human potential and human dignity, then we must first change our current institutionalized views of human nature. Leon Eisenberg, a psychiatrist at Harvard University, has illustrated examples of this concern in an article in which he has stated:

> The planets will move as they always have, whether we adopt a geocentric or a heliocentric view of the heavens. It is only the equations we generate to account for those motions that will be more or less complex; the motions of the planets are sublimely indifferent to our earth-bound astronomy. But the behavior of men is not independent of the theories of human behavior that men adopt.[11]

Although our biology has provided us with the ability to be human through our conscious abilities, culture is needed to provide symbolic information to give meaning to our conscious experiences. In order for meaning, symbolically imparted, to lead to human survival and to humane values, our cultural images of human nature must correspond to the reality of our biological being. Human values cannot be maintained in ignorance or defiance of our biology. The universe is run by natural forces, not by moral laws ("molecules do not have morals"). However, human societies, which obviously live in the natural world, must live by moral values. If these moral values contradict or ignore the natural laws, it will be the human societies, not the physical universe, that will suffer the consequences of such defiance. In an editorial comment on Henry Bent's poem "Necessary Ethic," the following was stated:

> It is said that there is a clear distinction between natural and human laws. Natural laws always hold; they are descriptive, while human laws can be broken; they are prescriptive. But the two kinds of laws are not totally separate—human laws must not demand the physically impossible; they must recognize and be based on the laws of nature that cannot be broken. Human laws also tend to be overthrown if they go too much against human nature—if they are inhuman or grossly unreasonable. . . . So the "Is" and the "Ought" aren't as clearly separable as a neat classifying mind might wish.[12]

It should be apparent that Western cultures are now applying powerful technologies within a Judeo-Christian image of human beings.[13] This view, arrogant and dangerous, portrays us as "superior to nature" and as "holding dominion over land and animals."

When one reflects on the philosophical options we have for ourselves, for our children, and for the future of the human species, I suggest that there are three alternatives: cultural absolutism or monism; cultural laissez-faire; and cultural bioethical pluralism. We increase our chances for the repression of individual human potential and dignity, as well as diminish our chances for survival, if we opt for either an "etched in stone"—absolute set of values based on a single view—or a "do your own thing"—laissez-faire attitude. Jacob Bronowski described this dilemma when he stated that "the problem of values arises when men try to fit together their need to be social animals with their need to be free men."[14]

We must accept the fact that our biological-historical background shapes in each of us unique, individual needs, while at the same time, we must realize that no human being could be human without other human beings. These specific biological facts of life should temper a sense of moral and social responsibility with other human beings and the ecosystem, as well as develop the individual sense of unique "selfhood."[15]

It seems ironic that in this era, powerful religious, economic, and political ideologies continue to support one or the other side of the nature versus nurture debate. Why has not the nature *and* nurture concept (which is the philosophical extension of the Mendelian and Watson-Crick theories of genetics) made its way into meaningful cultural, religious, political, and economic symbols? Are we, as members of a culture dedicated to technological intervention, going to continue to ignore the cultivation of scientifically sound views of human nature?

We may have criticized Chairman Mao for imposing one view on all the Chinese (suppressing individual uniqueness); however, we ought not to take pride in our cultural position. Our culture has gone to the opposite extreme, where social responsibility (being held accountable for the short- and long-term consequences of individual actions) is not rewarded. Whereas, in a symbolic sense, China could be viewed as a restaurant serving only one bland entrée to all its customers, the technological West can be viewed as a cafeteria that serves an overwhelming variety of stale and unnutritious, if not poisonous, food. We are what culture imprints on our consciousness and biology. If we are dissatisfied with human behavior, we need not blame biology, but rather we need only realter our cultural image of our nature so that it conforms to our biological limitations and potentials.

Science has provided several complementary models of human nature that conflict, in total or in part, with most traditional philosophical or theological concepts of human nature (Taoism might be an exception).[16] Until we take into account (a) the role of nature and nurture;[17] (b) the hierarchical relationship between the natural systems that are a part of human biology;[18] (c) the biocybernetic aspect of human behavior;[19] (d) the role of culture[20] on the forces of biocultural evolution,[21] we will only continue to exacerbate our psychological, ecological, and moral dilemmas.

NATURE AND NURTURE MODEL OF HUMAN NATURE

Presently, our culture has conflicting views of human nature as foundations for many social practices and policies. These views, having found their way into political ideologies, have shaped tragic, ineffective and/or inhumane policies in penal, medical, educational, and welfare practices.

Since all human traits, whether they are the number of digits on the hand or the ability to think, are the reciprocal products of gene-environmental interaction, it is imperative that all of us who are human intervenors internalize the concept of nature *and* nurture. Nature versus nurture concepts ignore the scientific facts that (a) genetic information has to express itself with environmental modulation and (b) that human beings have genes that shape the biological matrix on which environmental factors interact. Leon Eisenberg's statement accurately describes this model:

> By definition, the "genetic potential" for those traits will have existed in the individuals who exhibited them. But the translation of that genetic potentiality into the visible phenotypes occurred in a complex interaction with the physical and social environment that coincided with their evolution.[22] (See fig. 1.)

A specific example that illustrates the nature and nurture model may be seen in the human syndrome known as xeroderma pigmentosum.[23] At conception these individuals inherited genes that are unable to make enzymes (molecules catalyzing essential chemical reactions in the cell) that repair ultraviolet light-induced damage in the genes (DNA molecules) of the skin cells. These unrepaired, damaged DNA molecules in xeroderma cells then can lead to mutations, some of which presumably can cause carcinogenic transformation of the cell. If these individuals could be put in an ultraviolet light-proof environment immediately at birth (also in an environment devoid of ultraviolet-mimicking chemicals), then conceivably they would not contract skin cancers. In principle, for every genetically inhibited enzymatic function one could find an environmentally inhibited enzyme function. This is indeed what happens when "normal" persons, who have genes to repair ultraviolet light-induced DNA damage, are exposed to high amounts of environmental stress (in this case, massive amounts of ultraviolet light). This environmental stress overwhelms the ability of "normal" individuals to repair their damage. As a result, people who repeatedly get massive amounts of ultraviolet light have a higher probability of getting cancer than those people who are not exposed to sunlight.

This nature and nurture model underlies the fallacy of trying to examine any human characteristic from only a genetic or environmental perspective. Genes can only express themselves

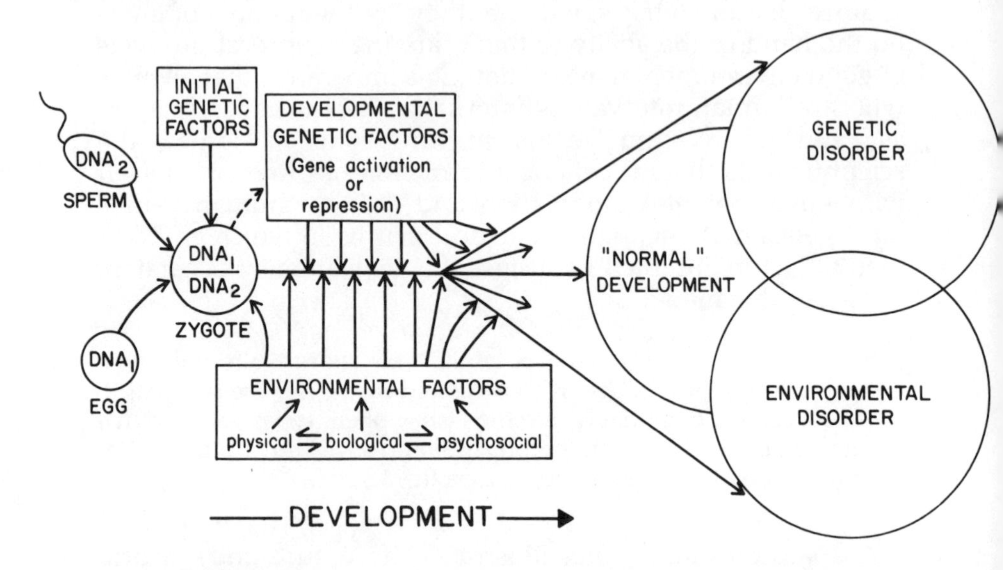

FIG. 1. Relationship between genetic and environmental information during human development, illustrating that the genetic information locked in the DNA molecules of the zygote must constantly interact with various environmental factors throughout development. Development will be normal or abnormal depending on either or both genetic or environmental predispositions.

in particular environments. Environments will alter the full range of expression of genes. Furthermore, environmental factors interact with a biological being whose matrix (flesh and blood) determine the nature of that interaction (e.g., photons of light with eye pigments of a normal or colorblind individual).

Much of the sense of bankruptcy attributed to modern medicine[24] results from the failure of the philosophical basis for Western medicine to take into account this nature and nurture view of human nature.[25] The resistance of microorganisms to "wonder" drugs, the resistance and susceptibility of individuals to various environmental triggers of various disease states, and the inability of the medical strategy, based on the germ theory, to conquer the chronic diseases are all the result of the failure to understand the delicate interplay between specific genes and the various environmental factors.[26]

This nature and nurture model allows us to see that (1) "normal" development is, in part, arbitrarily and subjectively defined by individuals and culture; (2) deviation from the "norm" can be primarily the result of a genetic predisposition (i.e., the skin cancers of a xeroderma pigmentosum patient exposed to a "normal" amount of sunlight) or of an environmental stress (i.e., skin cancer of a "normal" individual exposed to excessive amounts of sunlight); (3) intervention with technological *means* can, in principle, be through environmental engineering (i.e., placing sun-sensitive xeroderma pigmentosum patients in a sun-free environment) or genetic engineering (if and when it becomes available); and (4) the *ends* to which either of these *means* are shaped, in part, is determined by our understanding of what is implied to us when we state that an individual's phenotype is "normal."

To illustrate how questions like "Is cancer hereditary?" are reflections of an erroneous concept of phenotype, one can reexamine the xeroderma pigmentosum example and try to answer the question "Did the genes or the sunlight *cause* the cancer?" It should be obvious that the question is meaningless from the standpoint of traditional concepts, whereas the nature and nurture model allows one to see that the cancer was the result of the *interaction* of specific genes with specific environmental agents.

BIOSYMBOLIC OR BIO-PSYCHOSOCIAL VIEW OF HUMAN NATURE

This concept of human nature refers to the biological basis of human consciousness that creates a psychological need to explain our experiences. Culture, through symbolic language and mythologies in the form of social practice, gives meaning to our lives. In other words, the biological bases of maleness or femaleness, for example, are supplemented with cultural concepts for manhood and womanhood. If a culture's mythologies repress the biological forces affecting human nature, then the human potential is stifled. Students of social intervention must ensure that social practices enhance rather than repress human potential.

The work of John Money on the psychosexual development of hermaphrodites illustrates the powerful role that culture plays in shaping one's concepts of "self."[27] In cases where careful psychological preparation is given to parents of a hermaphrodite, together with cosmetic surgery and hormone intervention at appropriate times during the child's development, the psychological concept of "self" of the hermaphrodite can override the contrary biological signals locked in the sex chromosome.

In essence, the genetic-based (or cosmetically transformed) morphological structures of the external genitalia ("maleness" or "femaleness") are the visual signals that elicit culturally shaped responses from a young child's social environment. These responses are organized in time to shape an internalized view of "self" in terms of culturally imposed views of "manhood" or "womanhood." In the case of the untreated hermaphrodite, an ambiguous series of responses is received that, predictably, leads to a confused view of "self."

It would be a natural extension of this type of example to predict that children reared in a culture, which J. Knowles has described as one that "lacks an ideology,"[28] will not only lack a sense of individual "selfhood" but also individual self-worth. Moreover, the development of self in nonwhites living in a white culture may be virtually impossible. "Blackness" is a cultural attempt to help the developing Negro shape a harmonious sense of selfhood that is consistent with the biological potential. E. Cassirer's statement that "man is . . . no longer in a physical universe, man lives in a symbolic (abstract or ideological) universe"[29] portrays this aspect of human nature. Pointing out how our concepts of human nature are nurtured by our culture, Gyorgy Kepes has explained that "we make a map of our experience patterns an inner model of the outer world, and we use this to organize our lives."[30]

HIERARCHICAL VIEW OF HUMAN NATURE

This concept of human nature views all of the complex human traits and abilities as the natural emergence of the organization of complex natural systems in time and space. For example, human consciousness, like wetness of water, is made possible by the proper organization of atoms, molecules, cells, tissues, and organs during development. In other words, studying brain cells or molecular components of a brain alone will not lead to understanding the phenomenon of consciousness, any more than will the characterization of oxygen or hydrogen molecules lead to our intrinsic understanding of wetness. Complex human traits such as consciousness, however, must not be thought of as "unnatural" simply because reductionalistic analysis fails to explain it.

Gunther Stent has recently implied that the methods of science have virtually run their course in the study of "man" because of severe intrinsic limitations.[31] Granting that there are biological and cultural limitations to all means of knowing (including the methods of science and "structuralism"), Van Potter[32] has challenged Stent's position and come to a different set of conclusions. As a necessary component of this hierarchical model, complex and higher order human traits are in constant feedback loops with their lower levels (see fig. 2). Only by this constant feedback of information is the complex organization maintained. If factors external to the hierarchy block the normal flow of information, such as the inhibition of hormones from cells to target tissues, then the human hierarchy will tend to break down. Examples of disruptions from higher to lower and from lower to higher levels are shown in figures 3 and 4. E. Laszlo, a systems philosopher, has described this model:

> First we are a collection of natural systems, living things second, thirdly human beings, members of a society and culture fourth, and unique individuals fifth.[33]

This model, together with the others discussed in this essay, might be used superficially to support a "Skinnerian"[34] and "sociobiological"[35] view of human nature. A specific feature of this hierarchical model, however, demonstrates fundamental differences: B. F. Skinner denies the reality of the human will or mind, and Wilson's sociobiological concept implies that the genetic information, which controls the potential of human consciousness and its influence on human behavior, does so directly. The hierarchical model, on the other hand, accepts the existence and reality of the human mind and will as *natural* emergent properties of the specific organization of all the subunits below it (brain tissues, cells, enzymes, and so forth). This hierarchical model denies the ghost-in-the-machine model of human nature[36] as well as other dualisms between mind and body or the individual and the natural environment. As a natural emergent entity, the mind-will (self-will) is also one of the determinants of behavior,[37] as well as a subunit (together with other mind-wills) in a higher-order entity (culture). The human

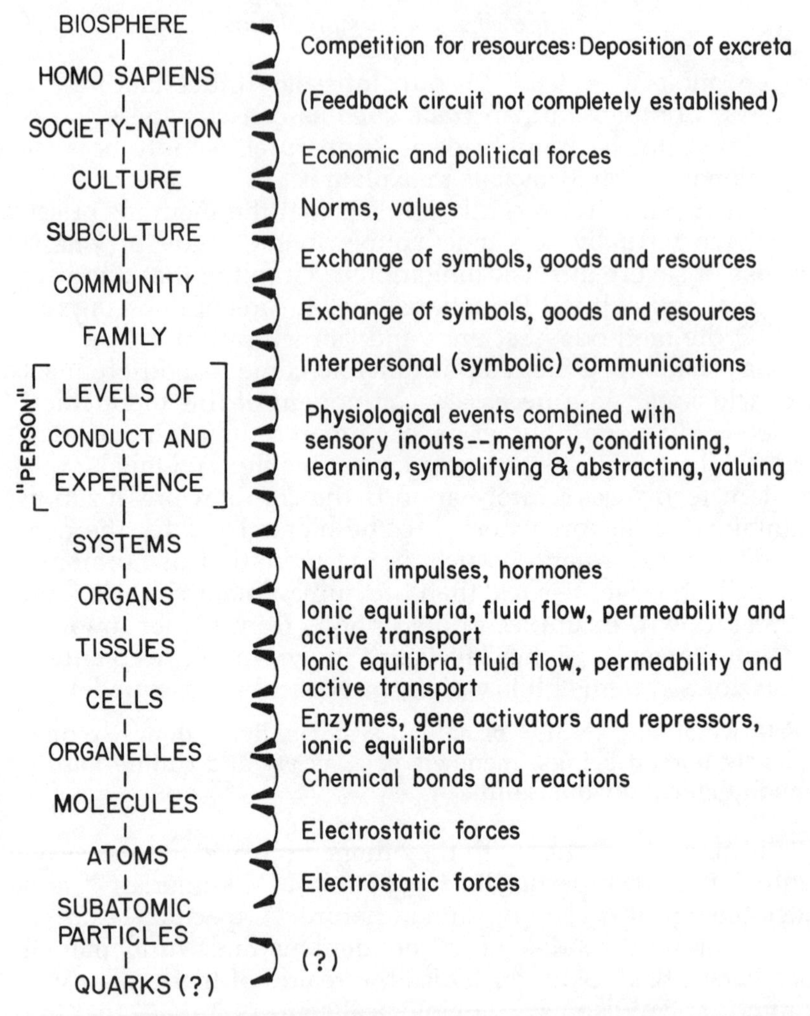

FIG. 2. Nature of feedback signals at various interlevel feedback loops in the man hierarchy. (Reprinted from H. Brody, "The Systems View of Man: Implications for Medicine, Science, and Ethics," ***Perspectives in Biology and Medicine*** **17(1973): 71–92, with permission of the University of Chicago Press).**

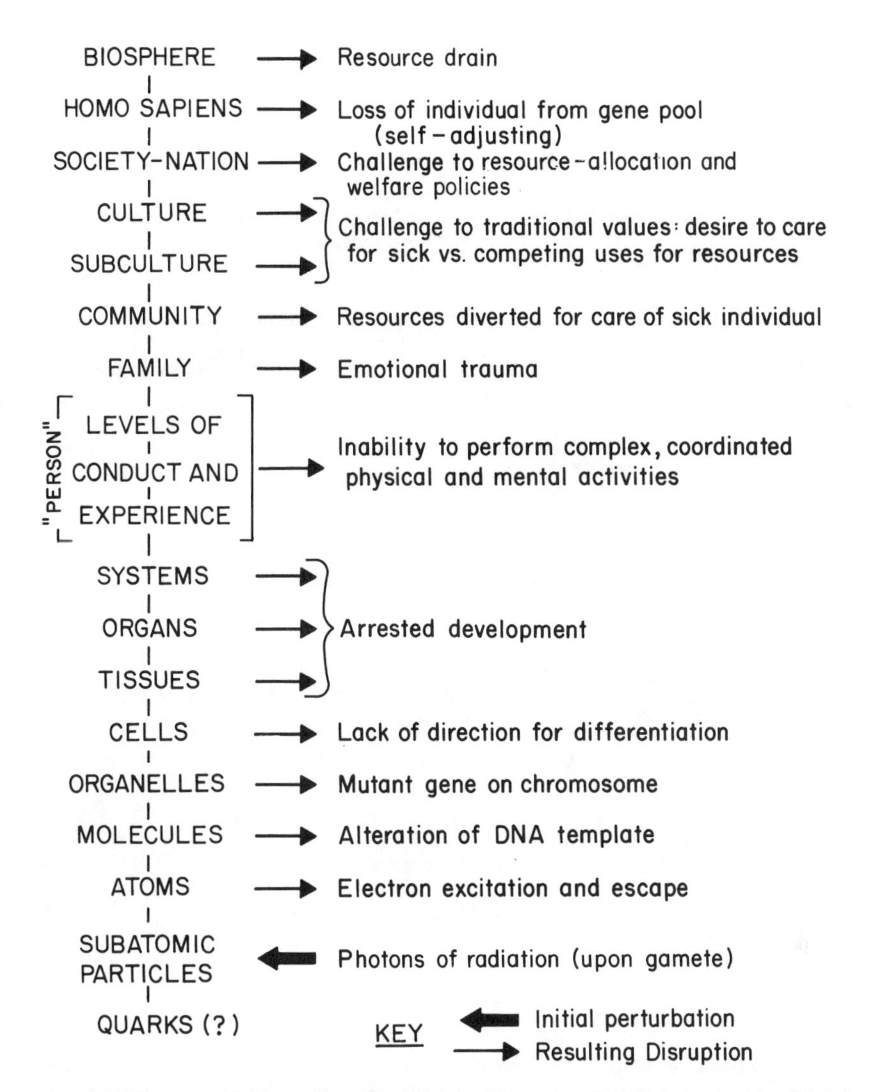

FIG. 3. **Disease example. Severe physical and mental retardation caused by a radiation induced mutation in the gamete: example of speed of disruption upward through the hierarchy. (Reprinted from H. Brody, "The Systems View of Man: Implications for Medicine, Science, and Ethics,"** ***Perspectives in Biology and Medicine*** **17(1973): 71–92, with permission of the University of Chicago Press).**

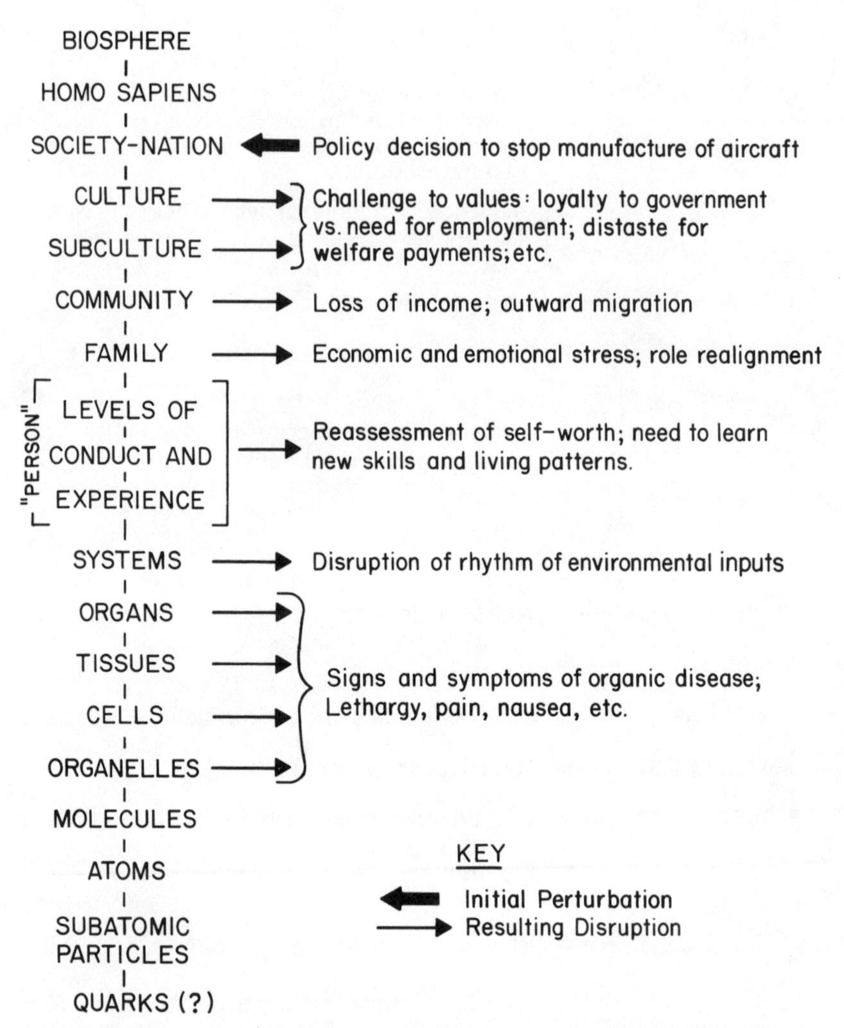

FIG. 4. Disease example. Stress-related psychosomatic illness in an unemployed aerospace engineer: example of speed of disruption downward through the hierarchy. (Reprinted from H. Brody, "The Systems View of Man: Implications for Medicine, Science, and Ethics," *Perspectives in Biology and Medicine* 17(1973): 71–92, with permission of the University of Chicago Press).

mind (an abstraction to describe a wide variety of conscious brain functions) is also subject to the factors described in the nature and nurture model[38] and the subsequent cybernetic model.[39]

CYBERNETIC VIEW OF HUMAN NATURE

The cybernetic view simply recognizes that human beings have control mechanisms that are based on genetic information and that regulate information from the environment (physical as well as social). This feedback of information is an adaptive biological process to regulate human output so that its effect on the human environment will not send lethal information back to the human being. For example, as shown in figure 5, human beings (as analogous to a thermostat) are the result of information input of both genes and culture.

Our unique human outputs, shaped by the input, have an impact on the environment in many ways. Examples of human output are biologically based processes of abstract thinking, symbolic communication, complex technological manipulation, and valuing. The complex interaction of these outputs changes the environment. The products of that interaction between the processes and the environment are historically unique ideas, symbols, technologies, and values. The social sum of that interaction could be conceived of as a definition of culture. The changed environment is the signal for new information that can positively reinforce or negatively depress these human processes. In essence, human beings cannot escape the consequences of their action because we are locked into the natural environment by this closed feedback loop. The freon-based spray device, for instance, is the end result of human abstraction, symbolic communication, technological development, and value decisions. This freon device has had an impact on human existence in both positive and negative ways. The changed environment of the atmosphere alone has had an impact on the physiological and genetic levels of the human hierarchy in that the destruction of the ozone layer by freon could lead to increased incidence of cancer by mutating genes in human skin. Perhaps Norbet Wiener has provided us with good insight for this model when he explains that "We have modified our environment (physical and abstract) so radically

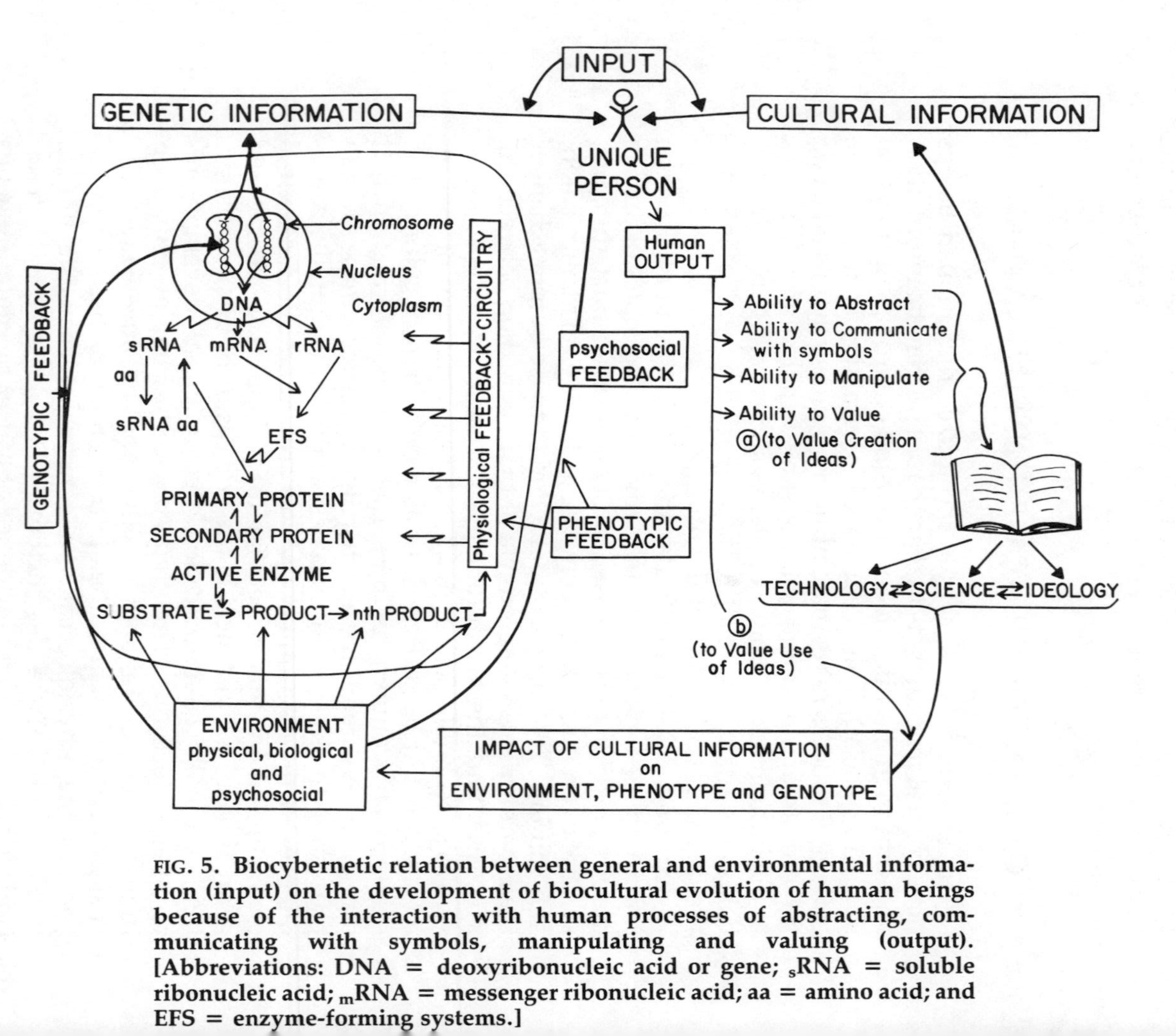

FIG. 5. **Biocybernetic relation between general and environmental information (input) on the development of biocultural evolution of human beings because of the interaction with human processes of abstracting, communicating with symbols, manipulating and valuing (output). [Abbreviations: DNA = deoxyribonucleic acid or gene; $_{s}$RNA = soluble ribonucleic acid; $_{m}$RNA = messenger ribonucleic acid; aa = amino acid; and EFS = enzyme-forming systems.]**

that we must now modify ourselves in order to exist in this new environment."[40]

This model helps one to understand how we, as human cybernetic machines, tend to behave in ways that are usually the result of the immediate—or shortterm feedback of information that allows us to feel the "goodness" or "badness" of our behavior. The longterm expected consequences of that behavior, if perceived at all (not all the consequences of our behavior are directly detected by our senses, as in radiation pollution), are only abstractions and are hard for many individuals to internalize. Consequently, the knowledge of impending feedback of negative or positive information is rarely a sufficient determinant of human behavior.

BIOCULTURAL-EVOLUTIONARY VIEW OF HUMAN NATURE

Human nature is the result of the interaction of a biological and psychosocial component. The psychosocial component, whose biological basis is responsible for human consciousness, shapes human cultures. Few would deny that human cultures change and evolve. What is usually not fully appreciated, or in fact, what is sometimes denied, is the biological fact that the human's biological basis is also subject to change (see figs. 6a, 6b, and 6c). Moreover, human cultures are creating new environments that are inducing human genetic change (i.e., radiation pollution) and selecting for, or against, old and new, simple and complex human traits. Unless students of human intervention are made conscious of this delicate balance between biological and cultural evolution, the human-shaped environment might ultimately prevent the potential of humanizing the psychosocial aspect of human nature. C. Fay has eloquently summarized this view:

> Consequently, adaptation on the cultural level involved an ethical system by means of which the social relations are organized. Whether the cultural system is in a state of equilibrium or desequilibrium will be of utmost consequence for the moral and social problem of individual human beings. In short, given a proper understanding of the human individual on the one hand and of culture on the other, it should be evident that there can be nothing

BIOLOGICAL EVOLUTION	CULTURAL EVOLUTION
L.C.D. = DNA Molecule	L.C.D. = Idea
DNA Properties	Idea Properties
1. Information	1. Information
2. Replication	2. Replication
3. Mutation: Copy-Error	3. Mutation: Copy-Error
4. Expression	4. Expression
5. Feedback	5. Feedback

FIG. 6a. Analogous properties of biological and cultural evolution. L.C.D. = least common denominator.

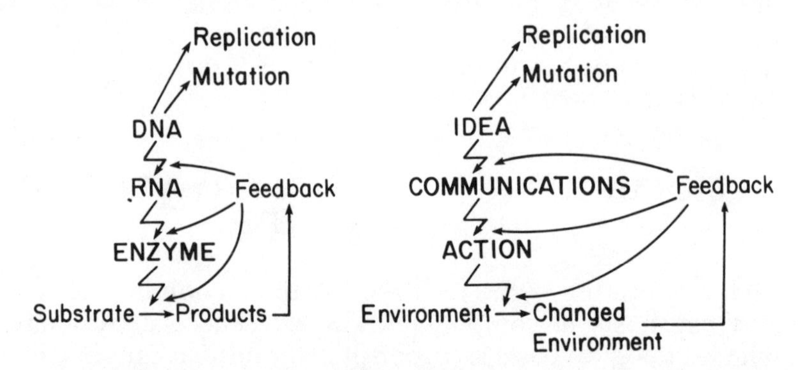

FIG. 6b. Flow of information and feedback in biological and cultural evolution. (Reprinted from Van Rensselaer Potter's *Bioethics: Bridge to the Future,* [1971], with permission of Prentice Hall).

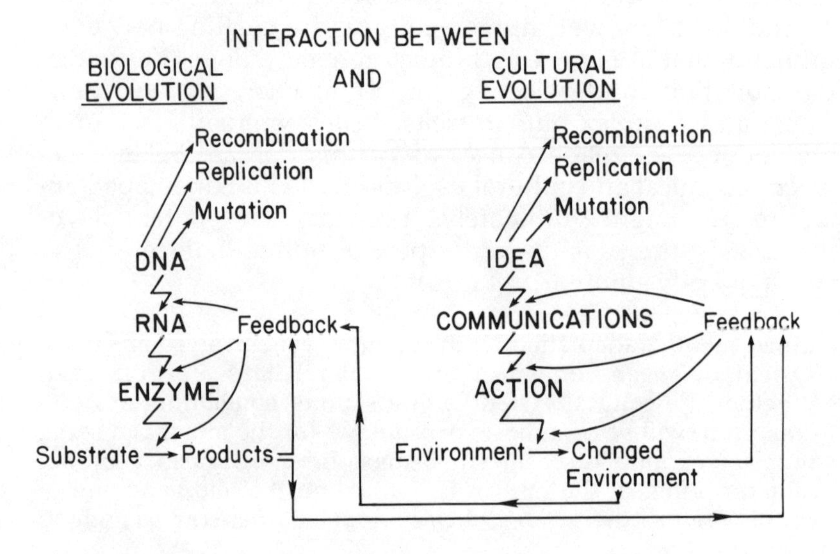

FIG. 6c. Feedback between processes of biological and cultural evolution (modified from Fig. 8.1, p. 107, in Van Rensselaer Potter's *Bioethics: Bridge to the Future*. New York: Prentice Hall, 1971).

> in the whole field of value, including that which is most private and unique, which transcends a biocultural view of the evolution of man.[41]

This model stresses the delicate balance between all the genes that need to work together to adapt to a specific environment and to ever-changing environments. The concept of stratified stability was developed by Bronowski[42] to explain this phenomenon. When we create with our human minds new environments in which the genes of our body are not adaptable, we are ignoring this important fact of human nature—our total dependence on, and integration with, the total environment.

OTHER VIEWS OF HUMAN NATURE

There are several other modifications of the aforementioned models of human nature, as well as additions to the list, which various scientific disciplines could contribute. For example, the probabilistic aspect, or the role of chance, of each of the five models ought to be noted.[43] Furthermore, explication of the biosymbolic or bio-psychosocial view could be made in terms of A. Maslow's self-actualization concept of human nature.[44] In other words, since human nature is the product of an interaction of biologically based impulses with culturally shaped rational interpretations of our experiences, evolutionary development of the individual, as well as the culture, will change both our view of our nature and our values.[45]

Unless human nature is analyzed in the context of both a micro- and macrocosmic view of the physical world we live in, the concept of human nature will be necessarily incomplete. Unfortunately, for most human beings any possible relationship that might exist between the subatomic world and our human values is far too abstract to guide moral behavior in any meaningful way.[46] The same could probably be said for our view of ourselves in an expanding or steady-state universe. The probabilistic evolutionary theme, however, that unites concepts of the micro- and macrouniverse to the biological views of human nature is itself an important concept to develop, as H. Morowitz has emphasized:

> We have spoken of Darwinian evolution as a loss of innocence. Indeed, it can be argued that the combined impact of evolution and the second law of thermodynamics represents the ultimate in nibbling on the forbidden apple. For not only is man himself a part of nature, a naked ape in the current idiom, but he is a naked ape in a universe that is decaying to a homogenized nothingness. Any philosophy of man or any theology which is not adjusted to this particular loss of innocence is simply ignoring the intellectual scientific milieu in which modern man must function. . . . It is extremely important to realize the full impact of the preceding ideas, because for Western man, at least, they represent a sharp break in the myth structure that has sustained him for many thousands of years. Regardless of the mythological details, that was almost always an underlying assumption that man was something quite apart from the world in which he functioned, something special and unique from nature, and destined to rule forever. If he envisaged the end of the universe, it was in an eschatological sense which was itself centered on man and his eternal being. . . . One note of further interest is the claim by some environmentalists that the ecological crisis has arisen due to the failure of man to realize that he exists within nature. There is a cultural lag between the scientific realization and the social implementation.[47]

THE PONTIUS PILATE SYNDROME

With increasing development of new technologies, we frequently hear in many contexts variations of the questions "Aren't we trying to play God?" or "Who will decide?" Implicit in questions like these is the idea that human beings are trying to alter the destiny of human life, which has been predestined by some Divine Plan. It is as though there is only one future and that human beings are incapable of altering that future. Moreover, these questions imply that our cultural evolution has occurred without human decision or human intervention. In point of fact, we are human beings because we do make decisions and because we do intervene constantly to alter our destiny. In the sense that we constantly intervene to alter our destiny, we play God. That is part of our nature as intervening animals. Not to use our abilities to intervene is to deny our human potential. This does not mean we must always intervene with every new idea or technology (quantity of intervention). Nor does it imply that we are unable to shape the nature of our intervention (quality of intervention).

Many of these decisions have to do with altering our relationship or dependence on the natural environment. We intervene on many levels to minimize threats to our dependence on nature for food (e.g., agricultural technology), for water (e.g., building wells or dams), for health (e.g., instituting sanitary measures or using drugs), for protection against the elements (e.g., wearing clothes, building homes with heaters or air conditioners), and for aesthetic pleasure (e.g., creation of art).

All of our biological abilities of thinking, communication, manipulating, and valuing are also dependent on human intervention in order that they be potentiated. For example, without a human parent's or a culture's concern for the maintenance of our human qualities, a newborn human being could not, by itself, become human. Culture, through parents or parental surrogates, must not only physically intervene on behalf of the child in order that basic physiological and psychological requirements be met but also must intervene by teaching the young child to communicate with symbols. It should, therefore, be obvious that the types of interventions by individuals or by cultures shape the outcome of the subjects of that intervention. Our values also will shape both the types of the intervention and the consequences of the intervention. Until we realize that our ethical philosophy, which shapes our values of intervention (moral value), is related to the consequences of our intervention, we will continue to reap the result of ignorance and of an artificial separation between facts and values. There is a characteristic feature of technological intervention found in Western culture. I find the phrase "Pontius Pilate Syndrome" a very useful concept in helping us to determine ethical modes of technological intervention. The following remarks by W. Vogt should set the background for the explication of this concept:

> The modern medical profession . . . continues to believe it has a duty to keep alive as many people as possible. In many parts of the world doctors apply their intelligence to our aspect of man's welfare-survival and deny their moral right to apply it to the problem as a whole. Through medical care and improved sanitation they are responsible for more millions living more years in increasing misery. Their refusal to consider their responsibility in these matters does not seem to them to compromise their intellectual integrity. . . . They set the stage for disaster; then, like Pilate, they wash their hands of the consequences.[48]

In essence, we find that the philosophical reasoning found in the West (not based on the scientific models of human nature presented in this essay) allow one to commit the sin of Pontius Pilate. By unwittingly, or even altruistically, intervening with technologies, we, like Pontius, set the stage for longterm disaster, but find cultural (ethical) support for washing our hands of the consequences. In a more general sense, and using another set of contemporary terms, we find cultural and moral support for putting the plug in, but find little cultural support for the possibility that one of the consequences of putting the plug in is having to pull the plug out. It seems only reasonable that those who intervene (play God, put in the plug) are ethically responsible for the consequences (playing God again or pulling the plug).

One might argue that those who act as Pontius (those who are willing to put the plug in, but who are unwilling to pull it out) ought not to put the plug in in the first place. This simple rule of advice, however, will not resolve most problems of technological intervention, since time and space often separate those who put the plug in from those who are left with the decision to pull it out or to put more plugs in. This seems to describe the case where many diverse plugs were put in years ago that allowed us to survive longer while being exposed to more of the carcinogenic effluents of the technology that gives us affluence.[49]

We have not found that it was morally wrong to intervene with technology to control infant death. We seem, however, to deem it morally wrong to intervene with technology to control birth. To uncouple, philosophically, death control from birth control is to ignore the consequence of one form of intervention (i.e., the Pontius Pilate Syndrome) and to absolve us from our responsibility for the longterm consequences.

HUMAN AGENDA

As we all know, any society that hopes to direct its future through a democracy must rely on an informed electorate. If that society chooses technological means to achieve its ends, then it is obvious that we have an inherent dilemma. There is no human way that each member of this technological-democratic society can be informed on the plethora of technological and value options. Moreover, such a democracy cannot long survive if it offers a laissez-faire policy for technological decisions to be made. Obviously, this does not imply that totalitarian societies will be any better able to cope with technological decisions, for there is also a limitation on the amount a dictator (benevolent or otherwise) can be informed on each new technology.

To afford technologies the full rights of legal jurisprudence given to human beings in our society will surely lead to major disasters. In essence, we must now adopt the attitude that technologies are presumed to be guilty until proved innocent. How, then, does a society choose to control the use of technologies? In effect, how can we eliminate the sin of Pontius Pilate?

It should be clear that the continued use of powerful technologies either within a laissez-faire philosophy or within a singular ideological framework for shortterm benefits will lead to a nonadaptive situation. In order that society of any political structure deal with the consequences of the use or misuse of the explosion of new knowledge and technologies, it has the option (a) to stop the creation of new knowledge and technologies, or (b) to monitor the use of technologies after they are created but before they are used. In my opinion, we need to create more knowledge and technologies, not less. I believe, however, that we must now institute control mechanisms to assess the technologies before they are used. This means we must be willing to trade off progress for reduced chances of disaster.

In brief, I think we will have to institutionalize cultural means to have, first, technological assessment by specialists, representing a wide variety of disciplines of every new technology, and second, value assessment of the technological alternatives. Within this kind of framework it would be the task of the technological assessment group to communicate their findings to both the value assessment group and the electorate.

If we are to design a technological assessment model for dealing with ecological and human problems caused by the intervention into human life with technological means to meet a variety of human value-directed ends, I believe we will have to separate the task of assessing the technological merits of each new technology from the value assessment. For the same group to cope with the value assessment at the same time a technological assessment is made ensures a conflict of interest, by having those responsible for collecting data also responsible for value-clarification and advocacy. At present I am in favor of a model based on the separation of a technological assessment group, whose primary function is to provide multidisciplinary technological analysis by specialists from a value assessment group, whose composition is made up from a broad spectrum of laypersons and whose function is to examine the consequences of various value-options for the collected data.

To provide the philosophical base for human values to control the *means* and *ends* of a technological society, I believe we must use all the scientific knowledge bearing on the study of human beings to construct a new view of human nature. I make the assumption that each individual holds a view of human nature that shapes policies and practices of human intervention, which, in turn, influences biological and psychosocial development. We must attack the cause, not the symptoms of our present and pending problems. The cause, I propose, resides in our head in the form of a bankrupt philosophy of human nature.

With a scientific view of human nature (e.g., human beings are inextricably linked to the biosphere and must conform to the physical laws of the universe), I believe we can understand that there is a philosophical option to ethical monism and ethical laissez-faire relativism. This option is bioethics. Although bioethics relies on scientific knowledge, it does not assume that science can determine which values are right or wrong. It does, however, demand that human values not be maintained in ignorance or in defiance of natural laws.

Within bioethics, science and technology can contribute to moral resolutions on three levels: (a) creation of new options; (b) formulating, as best it can, consequences of these options; and (c) understanding our biological nature and the consequences of the different value choices. Bioethics forces us to explicate our values, and it helps us understand which values maximize or minimize human survival and the quality of life.

The purpose of explicating the scientific facts and theories of human nature, then, is to have all of us become sensitive to the alternative values that maximize individual potential and social responsibility, while at the same time avoiding values that tend irreversibly to tip that balance. A special pluralistic attitude should be the logical consequence of this type of program.

The aforementioned, nonmutually exclusive concepts of human nature ought to be included as the integrative force for the various disciplines. They must not be thought of as models in competition with each other, but rather as complementary to form a holistic view of human nature; nor should they be considered as a complete list of conceptual paradigms. These models ought to be used as a conceptual framework on which to hang the data concerning human development (from molecular biology to social psychology). They should force each of us concerned with various areas of human development to assess the knowledge we believe is important to communicate in terms of the models. If this is done in an educational setting, the student and teacher will not be overwhelmed with seemingly irrelevant data from molecular biology, sociology, or psychology. Evidence for any of the concepts of human nature will provide means for courses of action dealing with human intervention by examining the consequences of various values and by focusing in on those pluralistic values that will be consistent with our biological nature. This is particularly relevant for the education of the professional intervenor. Jean Lemee speaks to that issue when he writes:

> In an era of change and flux, where values and principles are easily discarded and ever new and different views sought after, does not this ancient wisdom offer us something very practical and refreshingly simple? Namely, that the essential task of education and of all professional activities is to help men discover themselves as Man, and to provide the guiding principles to direct their activities towards a fuller life. . . . A profession is the exercise of expert human action, requiring knowledge, care and talent, and, as such, in a limited world, it carries consequences that man must bear. Should its practitioners enlarge their views of themselves and of Man, liberate it from self-imposed restrictions, it may flower into a liberal art. Should they choose, on the contrary, to narrow it to ever more circumscribed interests, it could degenerate into an instrument of oppression and dehumanization.[50]

That science can contribute to an understanding of ourselves, and, therefore, to our choice of human values seems to be an outrageous view to many individuals. From this perspective, science not only is unable to perform this difficult task but also is the major cause, in and of itself, for most human problems. To refute this notion of the failure of nerve, without arrogantly claiming science as God, Roy Ringo has argued:

> Then there is the argument that science by its very nature—rigid, logical, mechnical—is inhuman and will make life unlivable. This argument is ignorant nonsense. Even the cold-blooded judgmental side of science is no more inhuman than intelligence, honesty and lack of prejudice are inhuman. Moreover, the cold-blooded side of science is only one half of it; the creative side is as hot-blooded as poetry, and the application of science as human (and humane) as we choose to make them. . . . In fact, our ignorance of *man* [emphasis added] and his place in nature should make us at least a little skeptical of everything except remedying that ignorance.[51]

Moreover, Hans Selye has pointed out that:

> We must not reject science just because knowledge can be abused, for science can teach us those eternal laws of nature that govern our body, our mind, our conscience and, consequently, our behavior. There is no other way to overcome the ideological chaos of our time, which is created by the ever-growing conviction that reckless egotism is the sole moral code, supported by unprejudiced scientific logic.[52]

In the sense that beliefs about our nature, which are dependent on cultural input, govern behavior, which is considered our moral output, the human mind, although superior in some respects to the computer, is still subject to a well-known principle of computer engineers—garbage in; garbage out. Unlike the computer, the human mind is potentially capable of self-correction by feedback of knowledge. Human nature has two interacting components: our biology shaped by genetic-environmental interactions and our culturally shaped consciousness. Human genetics makes human consciousness possible. Human consciousness makes possible an almost infinite number of cultural environments. Because the genetic component of human nature is rather limited in comparison to the conscious component, however, it is imperative that the cultural manifestations of our consciousness (which includes our ethical and moral concepts) take into account the aforementioned realities of our human nature. Consequently, it seems that we ought to be able, culturally, to shape religious, economic, and political symbols that would take into account individual human uniqueness, without neglecting our universally shaped biological need for social and moral interaction. It is now up to us to change the cultural image of our nature or to suffer the ultimate consequence of our arrogant, chauvinistic, and erroneous image of ourselves. In conclusion, it seems appropriate to reflect on the words of Max Otto, who proclaimed in *The Human Enterprise* that

> The deepest source of a man's philosophy, the one that shapes and nourishes it, is faith or lack of faith in mankind. If he has confidence in human beings and believes that something fine can be achieved through them, he will acquire ideas about life and about the world which are in harmony with his confidence. Lack of confidence will generate corresponding ideas. A man's opinion of mankind may seem to originate in knowledge of physical nature and society; I believe it to be derived from firsthand experience with his fellows. Consequently, the growth of active division among men in recent years has resulted in social ideologies, national and racial theories, conceptions of the world in which we live, all of which rest on the premise that as realists men must regard each other as natural enemies who must settle their differences by cunning and might. It is of the profoundest importance that we see through these disuniting verbal or intellectual precipitates to the experience of disillusion and suffering which caused men to lose faith in men, and started them on those courses of aggression which then divided them still more.[53]

NOTES

1. See Gilbert Murray, *Five Stages of Greek Religion* (New York: Doubleday, 1925).

2. See A. Tofler, *Future Shock* (New York: Random House, 1970).

3. See Robert L. Heilbroner, *The Human Prospect* (New York: W. W. Norton, 1974).

4. S. H. Nasr, "Between the Rim and the Axis," *Main Currents in Modern Thought* 30 (1974): 85.

5. T. Colwell, "Some Implications of the Ecological Revolution for the Construction of Value," in *Human Values and Natural Science*, ed. E. Laszlo and J. Wilbur (New York: Gordon and Breach Science Publishers, 1970), p. 252.

6. Philip Rhinelander, *Is Man Incomprehensible to Man?* (San Francisco, Calif.: W. H. Freeman and Co., 1974), p. 89.

7. Bin-Ky Tan, "A Chinese Conception of the Nature of Man," *Main Currents in Modern Thought* 31 (1975): 145–48.

8. Edmund Pellegrino, "Medicine, History, and the Idea of Man," *Annals of the American Academy of Political and Social Sciences* 346 (1963): 9–20.

9. Albert Bandura, "Behavior Theory and the Models of Man," *American Psychologist* 87 (1974): 859–69.

10. James Drane, "A Philosophy of Man and Higher Education," *Main Currents in Modern Thought* 29 (1972): 99.

11. Leon Eisenberg, "On the Humanizing of Human Nature," *Impact of Science on Society* 23 (1973): 214.

12. A. Bent, "Laws and Laws," *Chemistry* 48 (1975): 2.

13. See L. White, *Machina Ex Deo* (Cambridge, Mass.: M.I.T. Press, 1968).

14. Jacob Bronowski, *Science and Human Values* (New York: Harper and Row, 1965), p. 55.

15. See Van R. Potter, *Bioethics* (Englewood Cliffs, N.J.: Prentice-Hall, 1971). I am deeply indebted to Dr. Potter, of the McArdle Laboratory for Cancer Research (University of Wisconsin), for the intellectual nurturing he has provided me over the years.

16. See F. Capra, *The Tao of Physics* (New York: Random House, 1975).

17. See Leon Eisenberg, "The Outcome as Cause: Predestination and Human Cloning," *Journal of Medicine and Philosophy* 1 (1976): 318–31; H. Harris, "Nature and Nurture," *New England Journal of Medicine* 297 (1977): 1399–1400; E. Inouye and H. Nishimura, *Gene-Environment Interaction in Common Diseases* (Baltimore, Md.: University Park Press, 1977); E. R. Scriver, C. Laberge, C. Clow, F. C. Fraser, "Genetics and Medicine: An Evolving Relationship," *Science* 200 (1978): 946–52.

18. See H. Brody, "A Systems View of Man: Implications for Medicine, Science and Ethics," *Perspectives in Biology and Medicine* 17 (1973): 71–92.

19. See Van R. Potter, "The Probabilistic Aspects of the Human Cybernetic Machine," *Perspectives in Biology and Medicine* 17 (1974): 164–83; idem, "Humility with Responsibility: A Bioethic for Oncologists," *Cancer Research* 35 (1975): 2297–2306.

20. See C. Geertz, "The Impact of the Concept of Culture on the Concept of Man," in *New Views of the Nature of Man*, ed. J. Platt (Chicago: University of Chicago Press, 1965).

21. See R. Alexander, "The Search for an Evolutionary Philosophy of Man," *Proceedings of the Royal Society of Victoria* 84 (1971): 99–120.

22. Eisenberg, "The Outcome as Cause," p. 321.

23. See H. T. Lynch; B. C. Frichot; and J. F. Lynch, "Cancer Control in Xeroderma Pigmentosum," *Archives of Dermatology* 1 (1977): 193–95.

24. See J. G. Rabkin and E. L. Struening, "Life Events, Stress and Illness," *Science* 194 (1976): 1013–20; D. D. Copeland, "Concepts of Disease and Diagnosis," *Perspectives in Biology and Medicine* 20 (1977): 52, 8–38; G. L. Engel, "The Need for a New Medical Model: A Challenge for Bio-medicine," *Science* 196 (1977): 129–36.

25. See J. E. Trosko and C. C. Chang, "Environmental Carcinogenesis: An Integrative Model," *Quarterly Review of Biology* 53 (1978): 115–41.

26. See J. E. Trosko and C. C. Chang, "Genes, Pollutants, and Human Diseases," *Quarterly Review of Biophysics* 11 (1978): 603–27.

27. John Money, "Psychosexual Differentiation," in *Sex Research: New Developments*, ed. J. Money (New York: Rinehart and Winston, 1965).

28. J. Knowles, "Utopia or Dystopia in an Age of Confusion," *Perspectives in Biology and Medicine* 16 (1973): 199–214.

29. E. Cassirer, *An Essay on Man* (New York: Doubleday, 1956), p. 43.

30. Gyorgy Kepes, *The Origins of Science*, ed. R. Abler; J. S. Adams; and P. Gould (Englewood Cliffs, N.J.: Prentice-Hall, 1971), p. 3.

31. See Gunther Stent, "Limits to the Scientific Understanding of Man," *Science* 187 (1975): 1052–57.

32. Potter, "Humility with Responsibility."

33. E. Laszlo, *The Systems View of the World* (New York: George Braziller, 1972), p. 25.

34. See B. F. Skinner, *Beyond Freedom and Dignity* (New York: Alfred A. Knopf, 1971).

35. See E. O. Wilson, *On Human Nature* (Cambridge, Mass.: Harvard University Press, 1978).

36. See A. Koestler, *The Ghost in the Machine* (New York: Macmillan Co., 1967).

37. See J. Platt, "A Revolutionary Manifesto," *Centers Magazine* 5 (1972): 34–52.

38. See R. Bunge; M. Johnson; and C. D. Ross, "Nature and Nurture in Development of the Autonomic Neuron," *Science* 199 (1978): 1409–16.

39. See Potter, "The Probabilistic Aspects."

40. Norbet Wiener, *The Human Use of Human Beings* (Garden City, N.Y.: Doubleday, 1954), p. 46.

41. C. Fay, "Ethical Naturalism and Biocultural Evolution," in *Human Values and Natural Science,* ed. E. Laszlo and J. Wilbur (New York: Gordon and Breach Science Publishers, 1970), p. 164.

42. See Jacob Bronowski, "New Concepts in the Evolution of Complexity: Stratified Stability and Unbounded Plans," *Zygon* 5 (1970): 18–35.

43. See J. Monod, *Chance and Necessity* (New York: Alfred A. Knopf, 1971).

44. A. Maslow, *Toward a Psychology of Being* (New York: D. Van Nostrand, 1968).

45. See C. Graves, "Levels of Existence: An Open System Theory of Values," *Journal of Humanistic Psychology* 10 (1970): 131–55.

46. See H. Margenau, "The New View of Man in his Physical Environment," *Centennial Review of Arts and Science* 1 (1957): 1–25; R. Schlegel, "Quantum Physics and Human Purpose," *Zygon* 8 (1973): 200–220; J. Prigogine, "Can Thermodynamics Explain Biological Order?", *Impact of Science on Society* 23 (1973): 159–80.

47. H. Morowitz, "Biology as a Cosmological Science," *Main Currents in Modern Thought* 28 (1972): 151–57.

48. W. Vogt, *Road to Survival* (New York: William Sloane, 1948), p. 48.

49. See Trosko and Chang, "Environmental Carcinogenesis."

50. Jean Lemee, "Educating the Professional," *Main Currents in Modern Thought* 31 (1975): 88.

51. Roy Ringo, "The Justification of Science to Scientists," *Bulletin of Atomic Scientists* 31 (1975): 33.

52. Hans Selye, "Science and Conscience in Harmony with Nature's Laws," *Impact of Science on Society* 25 (1975): 5.

53. Max Otto, *The Human Enterprise* (New York: F. S. Crofts, 1941), p. 366.

The Sociobiology of Human Sexuality: A Progress Report

MICHAEL RUSE

University of Guelph

In 1975 the distinguished Harvard entomologist E. O. Wilson published a massive tome, *Sociobiology: The New Synthesis*.[1] In this work, drawing on empirical and theoretical studies that had been appearing with increasing frequency in the previous fifteen years, Wilson brought together as one integrated discipline the science of animal social behavior, considered from a biological viewpoint. As he himself admitted, in one sense there is nothing new about this putative discipline of sociobiology. Even in the *Origin of Species*,[2] Charles Darwin, the father of modern evolutionary biology, had considered problems of animal social behavior, particularly those in the Hymenoptera (ants, bees, wasps). In the century since the *Origin*, much more work has been done in this field—in recent years most successfully by the so-called ethologists, like the Nobel Prize-winning scientists Konrad Lorenz and Niko Tinbergen.[3] But with reason, Wilson thought that there had been rapid and significant developments since about 1960, both in empirical studies and in the creation of theoretical explanatory models. In the field and in the laboratory there had been gathering of much new information about how animals, particularly those of the same species, respond to each other: weaker with stronger, mate with mate, parent with child, sibling with sibling. Similarly, complementing these findings, the theory of the workings of the central mechanism of evolution, natural selection, had taken off in new and exciting directions. Hence the new synthesis, and the new name, sociobiology.[4]

Since Wilson's book appeared, I think it is accurate to say

that the sociobiology of animals has gone from strength to strength. Monographs and journal articles pour forth. It is indeed true that there are controversies and differences between sociobiologists, but this is what one expects and almost hopes for in a healthy science. The main point is that no one really questions the science as a subject, or doubts that, roughly speaking, the kinds of explanatory models being proposed are appropriate. To use popular terminology, the science of the study of animal social behavior has found its paradigm; it is normal science.[5]

Yet the term *sociobiology* conjures up thoughts of controversy, even today. Why is this? The answer, as is well known, is that many sociobiologists have not been content to stay with animal science, but have also applied their ideas to our species, *Homo sapiens*. Thus, for instance, Wilson concluded *Sociobiology* with a chapter on humans, arguing that many of his explanatory models throw light on human social behavior. Wilson's claim was that much human thinking and action is less a direct function of the environment and social conditioning and more part of our evolutionary heritage, our biological wiring. That is, human social behavior is controlled at the immediate causal level by the units of heredity, the genes.

As can be imagined, this position did not sit very well with many thinkers, particularly those of the extreme left, who abhor any suggestion that human society is other than a human artifact and thus impossible to remold along ideologically acceptable lines[6] and those in the social sciences who saw their status and livelihood threatened by rapacious biologists.[7] Human sociobiology was (and still is) attacked on grounds of having committed just about every sin possible or impossible. It was found to be racist, sexist, and a doctrine of the far right. It was called incoherent, mystical, unfalsifiable, and (not very consistently) false. No one, we were assured, other than a person committed already to human sociobiology on dubious nonscientific grounds, could possibly take the nonsubject seriously.

My own feeling, on reading the critics' attacks on human sociobiology, was an uncanny sense of déjà vu. Almost all of the attacks could have been replaced by criticisms made a hundred years ago of Darwin's *Origin*, and no one would have been any the wiser.[8] Yet Darwin's ideas obviously survived. Why was this? Simply and obviously they survived because

Darwin had something to say of lasting value. His work, flawed though it certainly was in some respects, illuminated an important area of physical reality and formed a solid foundation on which succeeding generations of scientists could work. When all the dust had settled, Darwin's ideas went on, not because the critics were right or wrong—in many respects they were right—but because Darwin himself had something worthwhile to say.

Now obviously one cannot assume that because someone is criticized this implies he has something worthwhile to say, although this is a big step up from being ignored. But the Darwin story does to my mind imply that, to use a slang phrase, the proof of the pudding is in the eating. If an area of science has real potential, then it will last through—despite a shaky or speculative start, and despite criticism, fair and unfair. I think this applies particularly to human sociobiology. It might have been speculative in the first writings of Wilson and other sociobiologists. Indeed, it certainly was. But if there is a kernel of truth there, then it will attract good minds, and before too long we will see the results—empirical studies and solid theoretical foundations. If there is really nothing to human sociobiology, then it will wither away quickly enough, without the critics' help. Bright young graduate students are not going to ruin their chances pursuing a mirage.

Only time will tell. But this does not mean that we are not entitled to a progress report. Already we may fairly ask whether, since the first announcement of human sociobiology, any significant advances have been made in transporting it from the realm of the hypothetical to that of the actual. We can hardly expect to look for a fully developed, well-established, comprehensive science. After all, the regular social sciences have been going for one hundred years, and they hardly offer us that yet. But we might hope that some advances in some areas of human sociobiology have been made. Seeing whether this is so is the aim of this paper, which is therefore in a sense a midsemester progress report on human sociobiology. Sacrificing breadth for depth, I shall not try to mention absolutely every possible recent contribution; rather, I shall concentrate on work on one very central, and I believe representative, area of human sociobiology: sexuality. What I want to assess is the current status of the sociobiology of human sexuality.

THE SOCIOBIOLOGY OF HUMAN HETEROSEXUALITY

Sexuality goes right to the heart of sociobiology and shows just why it is that the sociobiologists believe that they have advanced significantly on their predecessors. Natural selection states that there is a struggle for survival and, more important, reproduction, and that there is a constant winnowing or selection of those fit organisms with helpful characteristics, adaptations—these characteristics being under the control of the genes.[9] A crucial question, however, is at what level the struggle occurs. Before the coming of the sociobiologists most people, although interestingly not Darwin himself, automatically assumed that the crucial unit of selection is the species, the particular interbreeding groups to which organisms belong. The sociobiologists, however, have argued strongly and convincingly that the unit of selection is the individual organism. This means that all characteristics, including behavioral characteristics, must be seen as rebounding to the benefit of the possessor. Hence, if an organism is seen helping or cooperating with another, this must be (in a sense) enlightened self-interest, as opposed to disinterested altruism.

The reasons why sociobiologsts plump so firmly for individual selection as opposed to group selection need not concern us here. They have been discussed extensively elsewhere,[10] and, rather like Columbus and the egg, once one sees them they are readily accepted without much dissent. If indeed there be characteristics for the group, they are few and far between. Let us move immediately from this view of the workings of selection to its consequences for the evolution and maintenance of sexuality. Under a group selection viewpoint, sexuality is considered valuable to the group, and most likely the species. Thus, male and female are designed to fit harmoniously together so that they can become one (as it were) in the conceiving and, where necessary, raising of offspring. Individual selection, however, sees things differently. In a sense, males and females are antagonists. (Only in a sense—at the behavioral level, male and female might cooperate harmoniously.) Not necessarily consciously, males and females try to maximize their representation in the next generation, because this is what selection is all about.[11] But males and females do not start from similar positions, and these different starting positions dictate different reproductive strategies, or general behavioral approaches that males and females should take in order best to reproduce. Restricting ourselves to mammals, consider the different strategies, as noted by E. O. Wilson in his recent book, *On Human Nature.*

> The anatomical difference between the two kinds of sex cell is often extreme. In particular, the human egg is eighty-five thousand times larger than the human sperm. The consequences of this gametic dimorphism ramify throughout the biology and psychology of human sex. The most important immediate result is that the female places a greater investment in each of her sex cells. A woman can expect to produce only about four hundred eggs in her lifetime. Of these a maximum of about twenty can be converted into healthy infants. The costs of bringing an infant to term and caring for it afterward are relatively enormous. In contrast, a man releases 100 million sperm with each ejaculation. Once he has achieved fertilization his purely physical commitment has ended. His genes will benefit equally with those of the female, but his investment will be far less than hers unless she can induce him to contribute to the care of the offspring. If a man were given total freedom to act, he could theoretically inseminate thousands of women in his lifetime.
>
> The resulting conflict of interest between the sexes is a property of not only human beings but also the majority of animal species. Males are characteristically aggressive, especially toward one another and most intensely during the breeding season. In most species, assertiveness is the most profitable male strategy. During the full period of time it takes to bring a fetus to term, from the fertilization of the egg to the birth of the infant, one male can fertilize many females, but a female can be fertilized by only one male. Thus, if males are able to court one female after another, some will be big winners and others will be absolute losers, while virtually all healthy females will succeed in being fertilized. It pays males to be aggressive, hasty, fickle, and undiscriminating. In theory it is more profitable for females to be coy, to hold back until they can identify males with the best genes. In species that rear young, it is also important for the females to select males who are more likely to stay with them after insemination.
>
> Human beings obey this biological principle faithfully.[12]

According to the sociobiologists, what we see in mammals are significant differences in behavior and temperament between males and females. Males need to be aggressive, trying to push other males out of the way, and promiscuous. Females need to be more domestic, careful, and reticent in sexual encounters; they have nothing to gain and everything to lose by unrestrained promiscuity. Furthermore, according to the sociobiologists, we should see these crucial parts of the theory holding for human beings, and we do. It is, of course, recognized by the sociobiologists that there is a cultural dimension to the human experience, and that while culture is normally biologically adaptive, it can override and even go against one's biology. Wilson and other sociobiologists claim, however, that when we see males taking the aggressive, dominant, promiscuous roles, and females the more domestic roles, this is not simply a function of social conditioning, but of our biology. Within this framework, a whole book devoted to the sociobiology of human sexuality has been published: *The Evolution of Human Sexuality* by Donald Symons.[13] In order to show how successfully sociobiologists explain human social behavior, let me explain three points discussed in some detail by Symons.

First there is the matter of sexual arousal. Although some recent psychological studies have been interpreted otherwise, daily experience and scientific evidence implies that men are much more readily aroused sexually than women. The pornography industry exists almost entirely for men; indeed, some magazines for women that used to feature nude males no longer bother to do so. Even those that still feature nude males find their primary market among male homosexuals. Many researchers, particularly social scientists, argue that these male-female differences are created by culture, concealing a deeper reality in which males and females differ little, if at all. Symons argues, however, that the differences are much more plausible if interpreted as part of our biology, particularly given the anthropological evidence that it is males who are erotically excited by females, rather than vice-versa. Many preliterate societies allow males to openly parade around with their genitals in full view; very few societies allow women to have uncovered genitals. Those that do permit fully naked females have rules or customs prohibiting males from staring, or females from openly displaying their vaginas (e.g., as when sitting). Symons writes:

> Male-female differences in tendencies to be sexually aroused by the

> visual stimulus of a member of the opposite sex—whether this stimulus is a drawing, painting, photograph, or actual person—can be parsimoniously explained in terms of ultimate causation, although their proximate bases remain obscure. Because a male can potentially impregnate a female at almost no cost to himself in terms of time and energy, selection favored the basic male tendency to become sexually aroused by the site of females, the strength of such arousal being proportionate to perceived female reproductive value; for a male, any random mating may pay off reproductively. In other mammals, female reproductive value is revealed primarily by the presence or absence of estrus; that is by ovulation advertisements. But human females do not advertise ovulation, hence selection favored male abilities to "assess" reproductive value largely through visual cues. . . . Human females, on the other hand, invest a substantial amount of energy and incur serious risks by becoming pregnant; hence the circumstances of impregnation are extremely important to female reproductive success. A nubile female virtually never experiences difficulty in finding willing sexual partners, and in a natural habitat nubile females are probably always married. The basic female "strategy" is to obtain the best possible husband, to be fertilized by the fittest available man (always, of course, taking risk into account), and to maximize the returns on sexual favors bestowed: to be sexually aroused by the sight of males would promote random matings, thus undermining all of these aims, and would also waste time and energy that could be spent in economically significant activities and in nurturing children. A female's reproductive success would be seriously compromised by the propensity to be sexually aroused by the sight of males.[14]

Next, there is the question of sexual choice. Here Symons is very much in line with the thinking of other sociobiologists, including Wilson. Biologically, there is no reason to think that male and female strategies with respect to the ideal marriage or sex partner will be the same. Indeed, biology suggests the kinds of differences that are reported by anthropology and that hold in respects in our own society. For men, the ideal partner is one that, if fertilized, will have the best chance of conceiving and rearing fit children. This means that there is a premium on relatively young, healthy women, and this, in fact, is what we find attracts men. Conversely, for a woman what is important in a potential mate is not the ability to conceive healthy children—men do not conceive, and in this respect one man's sperm is much like another man's—but rather the ability to aid the woman and her children. This can be done both through the conferring of admirable hereditary traits and aid in child-rearing (which could be direct or indirect). All of this adds up to the fact that age is not the crucial factor for the choice of men, but status is. Moreover, "from the female's point of view, a high-status male is both the best choice for a husband and for a sex partner."[15] Once having got herself a winner, a woman's best bet usually is to stay with him. Adultery for her pays only if she can upgrade the genes her offspring receive, or if (on a more permanent basis) she can get better child-care or help.

Incidentally, in the different male and female sexual strategies we see also the reason why polygyny (one man with multiple wives) is fairly common but polyandry (one woman with multiple husbands) is very rare in human societies. It can be in a woman's reproductive interests to share with other women a high-status male, whereby a high-status male in this context means a male with sufficient power and wealth to better assist the well-being of his close relatives and descendants than the average male. Marrying a man who already has a wife (wives) and is doing well has the advantage that one is going with a proven winner. Better to share a high-status male than to have a low-status male all to oneself. On the other hand, normally there is little advantage for a male if he shares a mate with other males; he is liable to spend most of his time and effort raising other people's children. (In a polygyny situation a wife will be putting an effort into raising children that she knows are her own). Hence, for the unattached male, rather than sharing a wife a better strategy is to find a wife of one's own, or to inseminate someone else's wife.

Finally, let me mention Symons's discussion of copulation as a female service. Both males and females enjoy sex. If anything, women have the capacity to enjoy it more than men, because they can have multiple orgasms in the same bout of sexual intercourse. Yet it is nearly always men—and rarely women—who have to beg and ask for sex, and to give bribes or presents. Prostitutes exist almost exclusively for men. Indeed, the two exceptions to this generalization go a long way toward proving the rule. On the one hand, we have male prostitutes for male homosexuals, as the advertisement columns of the biweekly homosexual newspaper, the *Advocate*, amply attest. There is no demand for (and hence no advertisements by) female prostitutes for lesbians. On the other hand, we have gigolos, young men who make a living servicing lonely, rich old ladies. But these men exist precisely because their patrons have entirely lost their female charms—looks and youth. Here and only here the imbalance between the sexes has swung the other way.

Why this uni-directional relationship should exist has often puzzled anthropologists, who think it somewhat arbitrary and inconsequential.[16] Symons's argument is that there is nothing at all arbitrary and inconsequential here. The one-way flow of gifts and requests stems from biology.

> Copulation as a female service is easily explained in terms of ultimate causation: since the minimum male parental investment is almost zero, males stand to benefit from copulating with any fertile female (if the risk is low enough), whereas females do not stand to benefit reproductively from copulating with many males no matter what the risk is.[17]

In other words, man's begging or giving payment for sex and woman's being begged or accepting payment for sex is a simple consequence of the unequal biological costs of sex. It costs a man virtually nothing; it can cost a woman a great deal. It is, consequently, in a woman's biological interests to be cautious and to expect some returns to help redress the balance. Payment is not simply a question of a crude dominant male corrupting an innocent woman with filthy lucre (or its equivalent).

THE MATTER OF EVIDENCE (HETEROSEXUALITY)

Human sociobiology continues to be controversial. Symons's book has been subjected to withering critical attack by the social scientist Clifford Geertz: "The moral equivalent of fast-food, Symons's book is not artlessly neutral, it is skillfully impoverished."[18] But my primary concern is not with the insecurities of social scientists; rather, it is with the truth-status of human sociobiology. What we want to know is whether there is any reason (or reasons) to take the sociobiology of human sexuality seriously. If there is, then we can discount all the suggestions that the subject is unfalsifiable or morally offensive. For instance, if women really do suffer from penis envy, then Freud is hardly a sexist in pointing this out; and if women really are domestic because of their genes, then sociobiologists are hardly sexist for pointing this out. On the other hand, if there is still no good reason to take the sociobiology of human sexuality seriously, then the critical attack starts to look a little redundant. It is full of sound and fury, but perhaps it signifies nothing.

We must be reasonable here. One can hardly ask for full well-confirmed theory, and obviously we shall hardly get this. What we need to show is that there is a body of evidence in favor of the sociobiology of human sexuality, and that taken as a whole it makes the enterprise a body of plausible hypothesis.

I believe that there are three possible sources that might incline us to take the sociobiology of human heterosexuality seriously. First, there is the fact that the sociobiology of human sex does not stand on its own; it is part of sociobiology, and specifically the sociobiology of animal sex. Sociobiology in turn does not stand on its own; it is part of evolutionary theory. Evolutionary theory is a well-confirmed theory.[19] It is reasonable to assume that, in general, organic characteristics are a function of genes that have been selected for their ability to confer reproductive fitness on their possessors. Moreover, that part of evolutionary theory which has to do with the social behavior of animals, sociobiology in general, is becoming increasingly plausible. I do not claim that it is all well confirmed or that all controversies are gone—they are not—but I do claim that there is increasing evidence that animal social behavior is under the control of the genes, and that the kinds of models sociobiologists propose are appropriate tools for explanation. In particular, in the case of heterosexuality it does make sense to consider the two sexes separately and to think that different reproductive strategies follow from the different contributions of males and females—in the mammals particularly, females being bound to take the more cautious approach in sexual encounters because they are the ones who take the brunt of the child-rearing (in most mammals, all the child-rearing).[20]

Do not misunderstand me. I am not trying surreptitiously to slip over the sociobiology of human heterosexuality. The whole point about human beings is that we have culture, which allows us to transmit ideas and attitudes at a level above the genes, so to speak. What I am claiming is that the animal sociobiology of sex works (i.e., has plausible theories). I also want to point out that human beings obviously have been subject to sexually dimorphic selective forces at the physical level—for example, the adaptive value of woman's broader hips—and that the physiology of humans (for instance, the difference in the sizes between the male and female reproductive contributions) is such that sociobiological factors could work. As pointed out above, human social behavior is what sociobiology would lead one to expect.

These factors do not make the human sociobiology of heterosexuality true, but they do start to lift it above the level of the ridiculous, particularly given that much social conditioning (e.g., Judeo/Christian religious moralizing) is designed to take us from what biology predicts, although many are unmoved. Even in Puritan New England adultery was not unknown, and every other repressive society has had its Hester Prynnes. I am not claiming that culture has no effect; obviously it does. The question is whether it has total effect. Selection can work even if a gene only manifests itself occasionally.

The second possible area of support for the sociobiology of human heterosexuality lies in direct analogies with other animals, particularly the higher primates. Wilson thinks that there is some support here. He writes:

> Characters are considered conservative if they remain constant at the level of the taxonomic family or throughout the order Primates, and they are the ones most likely to have persisted in relatively unaltered form into the evolution of *Homo*. These conservative traits include aggressive dominance systems, with males generally dominant over females, scaling in the intensity of responses, especially during aggressive interactions; intensive and prolonged maternal care, with a pronounced degree of socialization in the young; and matrilineal social organization. This classification of behavioral traits offers an appropriate basis for hypothesis formation. It allows a qualitative assessment of the probabilities that various behavioral traits have persisted into modern *Homo sapiens*.[21]

On the other hand, Wilson himself admits that one really cannot get too much from the primates. Among them one finds monogamy, polygamy, pair bonding, no pair bonding, male involvement in parental care, no male involvement in parental care, and most of the other options that spring to mind. Obviously, any analogies one can draw are more of heuristic value than justificatory. Significantly, Symons, who is a primate biologist, is very dubious about the value of analogies from the apes to humans: "Talk of why (or whether) humans pair-bond like gibbons strikes me as belonging to the same realm of discourse as talk of why the sea is boiling hot and whether pigs have wings."[22] Certainly Symons does not deny primate analogies entirely—he uses the chimpanzee as a model for our ancestors—but it is probably best to agree with him that we should not really look to the great apes for much support for the sociobiology of human heterosexuality.

Third, we have the question of implications and predictions that follow from or can be made on the basis of the sociobiology of human sexuality. Copernicus's theory was much more plausible after Galileo predicted and discovered the phases of Venus;[23] Darwin's theory similarly gained credibility after Bates's work on mimicry.[24] Can sociobiology yield analogous predictions about human sexuality, particularly those predictions and implications that are perhaps a little unexpected and hard to explain, especially if one subscribes exclusively to an environmentalist viewpoint? The sociobiologists claim that it can. There are two major pertinent predictions that have been claimed as following from sociobiology, but not from environmental theses.

The first prediction stems from the facts that one's psychosocial attitudes and behavior are linked to the nature of the brain and that, if sociobiology is correct, the genes of a man are going to cause a "masculine" brain and the genes of a woman are going to cause a "feminine" brain. If sociobiology is right, then no matter what the environment,[25] a masculine brain is going to cause male behavior and attitudes and a feminine brain is going to cause female behavior and attitudes. An environmental thesis implies that no matter what the genes, if one is brought up as a male, one will behave as a male (i.e., as a male as we now understand males), and if one is brought up as a female one will behave as a female.

Now suppose nature, with or without human help, plays a trick. Suppose that a person has a brain exposed to the kinds of influences one would expect from genes of one sex, but is brought up as a person belonging to the other sex. The environmentalist would expect the upbringing to be the decisive factor; the sociobiologist the influences on the brain. In fact, there are some people who do actually fall into the kind of class being supposed here. It appears that the genes of a male cause the fetal brain to be exposed to a higher level of male sex hormone, testosterone, than do the genes of a female (specifically between the third and six months of life, when the hypothalamus is developing). However, naturally and artifically, some females are exposed to the high testosterone levels during fetal growth. This means that they have "masculinized" brains. The sociobiologists claim that just as they predicted (and as the environmentalists would not have predicted), such genetic females grow up with male-type behavior even though physically they may be female and have always been treated as such. Thus, Wilson concludes that "at birth the twig is bent a little bit."[26]

The second prediction concerns homosexuals. In the view of the sociobiologists (Symons in particular), if the environmentalist thesis is true, one might expect male and female homosexual patterns to converge. Male homosexuals, having forsworn the ultimate "masculine" objective, namely trying to mate with women, will have no reason to be locked into other common male patterns, like looking continually for fresh sex partners. Lesbians, on the other hand, will have no reason to be as reticent as their heterosexual sisters, and will tend more toward the heterosexual male pattern. But, in fact, we find that what happens in reality is what sociobiology leads one to expect. Male homosexuals, unfettered by the reticence of a female partner, are incredibly promiscuous while lesbians are anything but that:

> The existence of large numbers of exclusive homosexuals in contemporary Western societies attests to the importance of social experience in determining the objectives that humans sexually desire; but the fact that homosexual men behave in many ways like heterosexual men, only more so, and lesbians behave like heterosexual women, only more so, indicates that some other aspects of human sexuality are not so plastic.[27]

My own view is that the sociobiologists can rightly claim that these two implications help to make their position more plausible than otherwise. How one critic, Geertz, can claim that Symons's views on homosexuals are "at about the level of descriptions of the Irish as garrulous and the Sherpas as loyal"[28] is quite beyond me. In fact, since Symons completed his work, there has appeared the most comprehensive survey ever done on homesexuality, that sponsored by the Kinsey Institute, and it confirms absolutely the difference between male and female homosexuals. Males have vast numbers of virtually anonymous sex partners; lesbians are much closer to the heterosexual norm.[29] All in all, therefore, I would argue that a case has been made for the plausibility of the sociobiological interpretation of human heterosexuality. I would not claim that it is an absolutely true or well-confirmed theory, but, as I pointed out earlier, I am not at all sure that one is justified in asking for such at this point. What we need to see is that human sociobiology is moving on from its initial statements, and this it seems to be doing in the realm of human heterosexuality, and that the hypotheses seem plausible, and this I suggest they do.

THE SOCIOBIOLOGY OF HUMAN HOMOSEXUALITY

Human homosexuality has been a matter of keen interest to sociobiologists, because prima facie the phenomenon seems to run in the face of the whole sociobiological program. Homosexuals are apparently not very good reproducers. This is not because there is anything wrong with their sperm or ova, but rather because the sexual acts of homosexuals do not lead to conception and reproduction. However, the sociobiologists are Darwinian evolutionists and are committed to the basic premise that the behavior of organisms must be understood in terms of reproductive advantage. Hence, we seem to have a clash between the reality and the theory. Sociobiologists have suggested a number of explanatory models to resolve this paradox. Two of these models illustrate the general thrust of sociobiological thinking on this matter.

The first of the sociobiological explanations sees human homosexuality as a function of balanced superior heterozygote fitness.[30] Simply put, this is a genetic mechanism whereby genes, the units of heredity, can be kept in populations even though under some circumstances the genes can have bad biological effects on their possessors. In sexual organisms genes occur in pairs. If both genes of a pair are identical, we have a homozygote; if the genes of a pair are different, we have a heterozygote. Supposing we have two genes (Say A_1 and A_2), if the heterozygote (A_1A_2) is fitter than either homozygote (A_1A_1 and A_2A_2)—that is, if it has more offspring than either homozygote—then the different genes will be held in balance in the population. This is so, even if one or both of the homozygotes is so unfit that it never has any offspring at all.

The application of this mechanism to the phenomenon of homosexuality is not hard to see. Let us suppose that homosexuality is a function of the genes and that possession of two homosexual genes makes a person a homosexual (we ignore the possibility that these genes may have other effects).[31] Also suppose, however, that heterozygotes—that is, possessors of one homosexual gene and one heterosexual gene—are fitter than homozygotes for heterosexual genes; in other words, that by one means or another heterozygotes reproduce more than heterosexual-gene homozygotes. It then follows naturally that the existence and persistence of homosexuality is a function of superior heterozygote fitness; the super-fit heterosexuals balance out the unfit homosexuals. Moreover, if it be objected that sometimes homosexuals reproduce, the theory can easily accommodate this fact. All that is necessary for the theory to work is that homosexuals reproduce less than heterosexuals. In every generation we will get a certain proportion of homosexuals.

The second explanatory model for human homosexuality, that based on kin selection, takes us right to the heart of the most exciting of the new theoretical ideas of sociobiology, animal or human. We have seen that from a biological evolutionary viewpoint it is reproduction that counts, and we know also that the sociobiologists are committed to the thesis that it is the individual's reproduction that counts. Granting that it is an individual's reproduction that counts, wherein lies the essence of this reproduction? Obviously it lies in the passing on of the individual's genes, the units of heredity. Note that an individual is not going to pass on its own genes literally; in fact, it is going to pass on *copies* of its genes. This is the key fact behind the notion of kin selection, for remember that organisms are related to other organisms—brothers, sisters, cousins, and so forth—and that an organism will share genes with relatives in the sense that they have identical instances of alleles. In short, inasmuch as a relative reproduces, copies of one's own genes are being perpetuated. In other words, theoretically, under certain circumstances, selection could promote genes causing characteristics that make their possessor cut down or forgo its own reproduction, so long as those same characteristics make this individual an altruist towards its relatives, in the sense that the individual increases the relatives' reproductive chances. This is kin selection.[32]

There is actually a little more to the story. With the exception of identical twins, one is more closely related to him or herself than to anyone else. Hence, under normal circumstances he or she will prefer one's own reproduction to that even of close relatives.[33] Simple arithmetic shows that if by forgoing one's own reproduction one thereby, for instance, increases a sibling's reproduction by over 100 percent, it is in one's own reproductive interests to do so. More copies of one's own genes are thereby being transmitted. More generally, if k is the ratio of gain to loss in fitness and if r is the coefficient of relationship of benefiting relatives ($0<r<1$), then for kin selection to work $k > \frac{1}{r}$ (i.e., if C is cost, and B benefit, $C < rB$).

It is easy to see the temptation of a kin-selection mechanism for the sociobiologist when faced with a phenomenon like human homosexuality.[34] Let me refer once again to Wilson's *On Human Nature*:

> How can genes predisposing their carriers toward homosexuality spread through the population if homosexuals have no children? One answer is that their close relative could have had more children as a result of their presence. The homosexual members of primitive societies could have helped members of the same sex, either while hunting and gathering or in more domestic occupations at the dwelling sites. Freed from the special obligations of parental duties, they would have been in a position to operate with special efficiency in assisting close relatives. They might further have taken the roles of seers, shamans, artists, and keepers of tribal knowledge. If the relatives—sisters, brothers, nieces, nephews, and others—were benefitted by higher survival and reproduction rates, the genes these individuals shared with the homosexual specialists would have increased at the expense of alternative genes. Inevitably, some of these genes would have been those that predisposed individuals toward homosexuality. A minority of the population would consequently always have the potential for developing homophilic preferences. Thus it is possible for homosexual genes to proliferate through collateral lines of descent, even if the homosexuals themselves do not have children. This conception can be called the "kin-selection hypothesis" of the origin of homosexuality.[35]

THE MATTER OF EVIDENCE (HOMOSEXUALITY)

To the best of my knowledge, the balanced superior heterozygote fitness hypothesis is still very much a hypothesis, with the ad hoc air of something that has been proposed simply because it would be one way of generating less than biologically fit humans. Also to the best of my knowledge, there are no studies showing that over a number of generations the ratios and distributions of homosexuals to heterosexuals fit those that would be expected were a balanced superior heterozygote fitness mechanism at work. Indeed, I am not sure how many studies there are showing how biologically unfit homosexuality actually is, although according to the recent Kinsey study, there is some information that perhaps adds a little credence to this assumption.[36] Heterosexuals are far more likely to marry than homosexuals (for instance, among white males heterosexuals are almost four times more likely to marry). When married, heterosexuals tend to have more children. Of course, we all know that one does not have to be married to have children, but given Bell and Weinberg's additional data that heterosexuals seem more likely to have heterosexual intercourse than homosexuals, one is really not being too speculative in concluding that the subjects of the Kinsey study suggest that homosexuality per se is biologically counteradaptive.

One other area of possible evidence should be examined. I refer to evidence that might be expected to show whether or not homosexuality is a genetic trait,[37] although note that a positive finding only provides a necessary condition for the truth of the balance hypothesis. There are many ways other than through homozygosity for a recessive gene that a characteristic can be controlled essentially by the genes. One could have straightforward dominance of a homosexual gene.[38] Even if it were established that the pertinent causative gene is recessive, it has not thereby been shown that (as the balance hypothesis claims) the heterozygote has fitness over all of the homozygotes.

How could one hope to show that homosexuality is genetic? A promising direction of inquiry is provided by twin tests. There are two kinds of twins: monozygotic twins, who share the same genotype, and dizygotic, who do not and are, therefore, no more closely related than normal siblings (i.e., fifty percent). If one finds significant differences between monozygotic twins and the differences between dizygotic twins, then (since generally the environment of twins is the same for both) a reasonable inference is that genetic factors are involved. The results of a major study on homosexual twins are astoundingly impressive.[39] Kallmann's study of eighty-five sets of twins where at least one twin exhibited homosexual behavior showed that in *all* forty monozygotic cases both twins were homosexual (and, moreover, homosexual to much the same intensity), whereas in the dizygotic cases most of the twins of homosexuals showed little or no homosexual inclination or behavior. One could not ask for stronger evidence of a genetic component to human homosexuality. Indeed, the evidence is so strong that one is reminded of Mendel's too-perfect figures confirming his pea plant experiments.

Against Kallmann's study it must be noted that since his work was done a few cases of monozygotic twins with different sexual orientations have been discovered.[40] So it certainly does not seem to be the case that all homosexuality is absolutely fixed by the genes. These counterfindings suggest two (not necessarily incompatible) possibilities. First, there are multiple causes of homosexuality. Perhaps some forms of homosexuality are essentially a function of the genes; other forms (or manifestations) require a significant environmental input. The other possiblity is simply that at least one form of homosexuality has a genetic base, but still requires some kind of special environmental input. Without it, one is heterosexual. (Alternatively, some form or manifestation of heterosexuality might require some kind of special environmental input. Without it, one is homosexual.) It should be added that some of the reported counterexamples to Kallmann's study (i.e., monozygotic twins with different sexual orientations) lend plausiblity to one or the other of these possibilities, both of which demand some specific environmental input to produce homosexuality. In the reported cases there is evidence that the twins of a pair were treated differently, with the latent homosexual twin generally getting more mothering, being treated more like a girl (nearly all the cases are of males), and so forth.

All in all, the evidence from twin tests is fairly strong support for the belief that the genes may play some role in homosexuality, although studies show also that the environment plays an important role. This finding, incidentally, brings us full circle back to Freud, for this was precisely his belief.[41] As pointed out, this conclusion does not support the balanced superior heterozygote fitness hypothesis as such. The evidence is certainly compatible with other genetic mechanisms. I suggest, therefore, that this analysis so far has shown that quite possibly homosexuality (at least some homosexuality) has a genetic component in the sense described above; that it is highly improbable that the environment does not play an important role; that the environmental input might be connected to familiar factors like psychologically suffocating mothering; and that, while the balance hypothesis has not been proved false, it is unlikely to be the exclusive source of human homosexuality—indeed, its major recommendation is that it is one way to get reduced fertility (which it is assumed that homosexuals have).

Consider now the second hypothesis, which centers on kin selection. Applying this mechanism to homosexuality, one assumes that homosexuals reduce their own reproductive fitness in order to boost the fitness of close relatives, especially siblings. There may not be anything intentional about this, but the effect is that homosexuals become altruists toward close relatives because they thereby increase their own overall inclusive fitness. I take it that this explanation is genetic in that the homosexual potential exists, but is environmental in that it requires some reason to trigger it. One would want some environmental reason suggesting (not necessarily consciously) that heterosexuality would be a bad reproductive strategy. In this, the kin selection hypothesis differs from the balance hypothesis. It differs also in expecting the homosexual to be altruistic toward close relatives; close relatives must breed better because of the homosexual's homosexuality.

A number of sociobiologists have suggested that a major causal key to human homosexuality may lie in this theory of kin selection.[42] There are, for instance, many reports in the anthropological literature of homosexuality of various forms in preliterate societies. One gets various kinds of cross-dressing—that is, wearing the clothes of the opposite sex to achieve erotic arousal in members of one's own sex[43]—adoption of the customs of the opposite sex, homosexual liaisons (i.e., involving homosexual intercourse), and even in some societies certain forms of homosexual marriage. Unfortunately, many of the reports almost exclusively concern adults. This means that there is little information on whether something occurred in the homosexual's childhood that would have sufficiently tipped the balance to make adult homosexuality an attractive reproductive strategy. What information there is, however, suggests that taking the homosexual strategy does frequently follow, or is accompanied by, phenomena of the suspected kind. For instance, at one time among the Araucans of South America, all ritualized homosexuals "were men who had taken up the role of women, who took the passive role in homosexual relations, and who were chosen for the role in childhood due to their feminine mannerisms or certain physical deformities."[44] Among the Nuer, a "woman who marries another woman is usually barren. . . ."[45] Among the Toradjas, the male homosexual life-style and women's work occur primarily because of "cowardice or some harrowing experience."[46] Generally, ritualized homosexual roles seem "to be attractive to individuals who have undergone some trauma, regardless of whether this involves a change of sex,"[47] although there certainly are exceptions.

In our own society there is similar evidence. "In accounts of modern male-to-female transsexuals, it is very common to read of some sort of childhood traumas immediately preceding the appearance of femininity."[48] A study of a group of effeminate boys (who apparently have a much higher probability of turning out homosexual than do average boys) "showed an above-average incidence of certain physical defects."[49] Additionally, a careful study implied that there are fairly significant physical differences between adult male homosexuals and adult male heterosexuals. On average (i.e., there are definite exceptions), heterosexuals are heavier (although not taller) than homosexuals (13¾ pounds) and stronger. As a statistical ensemble, homosexuals "had less subcutaneous fat and smaller muscle/bone development and were longer in proportion to bulk. Their shoulders were narrower in relation to pelvic width, and their muscle strength was less."[50] Given the fact that there are fairly strong links between child development and the adult state, one might suppose that, as a group, future homosexuals contain the slighter, weaker children, and that, consequently for them, a homosexual strategy is the most attractive option from a biological viewpoint. Incidentally, lesbians tend to be taller than female heterosexuals. Would it make sense to suggest that this similarly is relevant to the calculation of most attractive sexual strategy?

So far we have considered only reasons why homosexuals might not get involved in heterosexual activity. There is also the other side to the kin-selection coin, and that is the expectation that homosexuals can and will aid relatives. Again starting with preliterate societies, we find that homosexuals of various forms tend to have high status, which would presumably redound to the credit of close relatives. In society after society certain members take up the roles of members of the opposite sex, dressing in such a way, performing tasks appropriate to their opposite sex, and engaging in relations with members of their own sex. Moreover, with very few exceptions, such homosexuals have high status within the societies because they are considered to have certain special magical or religious powers and act as priests or shamans. Thus, among the Western Inoits, "advice always followed"; the Araucans, "advice required for every important decision"; the Cheyenne, "goes to war; matchmaker; supervises scalps and scalp ceremonies"; the Illinois, "required for all important decisions"; the Navaho, "wealthy leaders; mediators; matchmakers; unusual opportunity for material advancement"; the Sioux, "extraordinary privileges"; the Sea Dyaks, "rich; person of great consequence, often chief."[51] In short, being a homosexual in such societies and taking on a homosexual role often led to very high status and opportunity to advance the cause and comforts of close relatives. That is, homosexuals were specially suited to raising the reproductive chances of those who shared their genes, which is precisely what is required for the efficient operation of kin selection.

Of course, in our own society it is hardly true to say that homosexuals as such have an elevated status; indeed, they tend to be despised and persecuted. But there does seem to be some evidence that homosexuals have special abilities which would fit in well with the roles that they would have been expected to play in preliterate societies, where the sociobiologists think that natural selection would have had its crucial influence. Indeed, the abilities might even be such as to raise the reproductive-aid capacities of homosexuals in our own society, despite their apparent low status.

For example, evidence shows that homosexuals tend to have

greater acting ability than heterosexuals.[52] Of course, it is well known in our society that the stage (and the arts generally) has a far higher proportion of homosexuals than, say, the teaching profession. Undoubtedly, this is at least partially a function of the fact that homosexuals are attracted to the stage precisely because they know that here they will be accepted as normal persons. There are also surely cases of heterosexuals who behave homosexually for the sake of professional advancement. However, homosexuality and a dramatic flair may have a more complex causal connection. For instance, effeminate boys (a group with proportionately more future homosexuals than average) "are unusually adept at stage-acting and role-taking—at an age long before they could know that the acting profession has an unusually high incidence of homosexuality."[53] In other words, there is at least the possibility of a genetic link between homosexuality and acting ability (that is, between some homosexuality and some acting ability). Obviously, possession of acting ability would be of value to a priest or shaman, given that so much of their work centers on magic, mysteries, and ceremonies.

Homosexuals also tend to have a higher I.Q. than heterosexuals. Several studies support this claim.[54] Of course, the whole question of "intelligence" and I.Q. tests gets into very murky areas, and some of the more grandiose and pernicious claims have been very properly criticized. The frequently expressed fear, however, that I.Q. does not really represent some absolute quality of brightness, but more an ability to get on in society (and to do well on things that teachers value, such as I.Q. tests), supports the kin-selection hypothesis rather than detracts from it. Raising children is apparently something almost anyone can do, although obviously some do it better than others. What homosexuals need to do, given the kin-selection hypothesis, is to raise themselves in society to such an extent that they can bring back benefits for their kin (e.g., having influence to find good jobs for nephews and nieces). In other words, they need to possess just those abilities and attitudes that critics fear are reflected on I.Q. tests. If society demands conformity rather than ingenuity, if the tests measure the former rather than the latter, and if homosexuals do better than heterosexuals on the tests, so much the better for the kin-selection hypothesis.

Considered as a whole, how convincing is the evidence for

the kin-selection hypothesis for human homosexuality? I would suggest that a case has been made for taking seriously the hypothesis that at least some human homosexuality may be a causal function of the operation of kin selection, if not in our own society, then in the societies of our ancestors. On the other hand, it is clear that as yet no definitive justification has been offered for the hypothesis. For instance, no proof has yet been offered showing that homosexuals really do raise the fitness of their relatives, and thus indirectly their own inclusive fitness. Is it indeed the case that siblings of homosexuals successfully rear more offspring than they would otherwise? It would certainly be interesting to know, even in our own society, what attitudes homosexuals have toward their siblings, nephews, and nieces. Is there evidence (e.g., in the form of money left on death) that homosexuals help their relatives? Similarly, much more work needs to be done on the nature of homosexuals themselves. Do we systematically find that personal reproductive capacity of homosexuals or future homosexuals is reduced? Again, the evidence is as yet hardly definitive. In short, the case for homosexuality seems not proved, but it ought to be taken seriously by anyone interested in the etiology of human homosexuality.

CONCLUSION

One swallow does not a summer make, nor even do two swallows, one hetero- and one homosexual. But I think now we are in a position to make an assessment of the status of human sociobiology as it stands at present. One point is certainly clear: no one could claim that it is a well-established theory. Most important, however, is the question whether, given its young age, human sociobiology has done all that might reasonably be expected. Do we have some new models, do they throw light on dimensions of the human experience, do they find a reasonably responsive echo of confirmation? My own opinion is that, considered with respect to the specific (but very crucial) topic of human sexuality, the answers to these questions are sufficiently positive to continue to take human sociobiology seriously, but no more. It has still a long way to go before (to revert to Thomas Kuhn's language) it can lay claim to being an established paradigm and its practitioners can consider themselves normal scientists.

NOTES

1. Cambridge, Mass.: Harvard University Press, Belknap Press.
2. London: John Murray, 1859.
3. See, for example, Konrad Lorenz, *On Aggression* (London: Methuen, 1966) and N. Tinbergen, *Social Behaviour in Animals* (London: Methuen, 1953).
4. For a survey of major sociobiological contributions, see my *Sociobiology: Sense or Nonsense?* (Dordrecht, Holland: Reidel Publishing Co., 1979).
5. See Thomas Kuhn, *The Structure of Scientific Revolutions*, 2d ed. (Chicago: University of Chicago Press, 1970).
6. For example, E. Allen et al. "Sociobiology: Another Biological Determinism," *BioScience* 26 (1976): 182–86.
7. For example, M. Sahlins, *The Use and Abuse of Biology* (Ann Arbor: University of Michigan Press, 1976).
8. For a discussion of the controversy after Darwin, see my *The Darwinian Revolution: Science Red in Tooth and Claw* (Chicago: University of Chicago Press, 1979).
9. In this paper I am trying to keep to a minimum the technical biology. Good introductions to the pertinent biology are T. Dobzhansky et al. *Evolution* (San Francisco, Calif.: Freeman, 1977), F. J. Ayala and J. W. Valentine, *Evolving* (San Francisco, Calif.: Benjamin/Cummings, 1979), and E. Mayr, *Animal Species and Their Evolution* (Cambridge, Mass.: Harvard University Press, Belknap Press, 1963). Alternatively, the reader might look at my *The Philosophy of Biology* (London: Hutchinson, 1973).
10. See particularly G. C. Williams, *Adaptation and Natural Selection* (Princeton, N.J.: Princeton University Press, 1966). I discuss Darwin's position in "Charles Darwin and Group Selection," *Annals of Science* 37: (1980) 615–31.
11. I am using teleological language here because biologists do. Less teleologically one might say that males and females have different genes, which give rise to behaviors that will, on average, be such as to lead to maximum representations in the next generation. I am not sure whether this is entirely nonteleological, or indeed whether a nonteleological way of describing theories is possible or useful.
12. Cambridge, Mass.: Harvard University Press, Belknap Press, 1978, pp. 124–25.
13. New York: Oxford University Press, 1979.
14. Ibid, p. 180.
15. Ibid, p. 193.
16. See, for instance, B. Malinowski, *The Sexual Life of Savages in North-Western Melanesia* (New York: Halcyon House, 1929).
17. Symons, *Evolution of Human Sexuality*, p. 261.
18. Clifford Geertz, "Sociosexology," *New York Review of Books*, 24 January 1980, p. 4.
19. Doubters should consult the works mentioned in note 9.
20. I discuss this in detail in *Sociobiology: Sense or Nonsense?* (note 4).
21. Wilson, *Sociobiology*, p. 551.
22. Symons, *Evolution of Human Sexuality*, p. 108.
23. Thomas Kuhn, *The Copernican Revolution* (Cambridge, Mass.: Harvard University Press, 1957).
24. Ruse, *Darwinian Revolution*, pp. 207–8.
25. That is, no matter what the naturally occurring environment might be. Sociobiologists would not deny that humans might manipulate the environment to bring about effects that never occur naturally.
26. Wilson, *On Human Nature*, p. 132. I might add parenthetically that the literature on hormones and sexuality is big and growing. Somewhat different positions can be found in J. Money and A. Ehrhardt, *Man and Woman, Boy and Girl* (Baltimore, Md.:

Johns Hopkins University Press, 1972), and G. Dörner, *Hormones and Brain Differentiation* (Amsterdam: Elsevier, 1976). Recent reviews occur in *Handbook of Sexology*, ed. J. Money and H. Muspah (New York: Elsevier, 1977). I myself discuss the matter in some detail in my *Homosexuality: A Philosophical Perspective* (Berkeley: University of California Press, 1982).

27. Symons, *Evolution of Human Sexuality*, pp. 304–5.

28. Geertz, "Sociosexology," p. 4.

29. A. Bell and M. Weinberg, *Homosexualities: A Study of Diversity Among Men and Women* (New York: Simon and Schuster, 1978).

30. This model was first proposed in G. E. Hutchinson, "A Speculative Consideration of Certain Possible Forms of Sexual Selection in Man," *American Naturalist* 93 (1959): 81–91. Obviously Hutchinson's work is hardly recent sociobiology, but one can justifiably discuss the model here because it and its evidence have been taken up by the sociobiologists, especially by Wilson in *Sociobiology* and in *On Human Nature.*

31. In this paper I assume a fairly strong connection between homosexual orientation and homosexual behavior, but I shall not discuss questions having to do with intensity or degree of homosexual orientation/behavior. A more detailed sociobiological analysis could consider these distinctions.

32. See W. D. Hamilton, "The Genetical Theory of Social Behavior," *Journal of Theoretical Biology* 7 (1964): 1–32; Wilson, *Sociobiology;* R. Dawkins, *The Selfish Gene* (Oxford: At the University Press, 1976); D. Barash, *Sociobiology and Behavior* (New York: Elsevier, 1977).

33. Not necessarily conciously. The genes program organisms to behave as though conscious preference were at work.

34. Wilson, *Sociobiology* and *On Human Nature;* J. D. Weinrich, "Human Reproductive Strategy" (Ph.D. diss., Harvard University, 1976).

35. Wilson, *On Human Nature*, pp. 144–45.

36. Bell and Weinberg, *Homosexualities.*

37. See D. L. Hull, "The Trouble with Traits," *Theory and Decision* (forthcoming).

38. Of course, the genes themselves are not homosexual. By homosexual gene is meant homosexual-orientation-causing gene.

39. F. Kallman, "Comparative Twin Study of the Genetic Aspects of Male Homosexuality," *Journal of Nervous and Mental Disorders* 115 (1952): 283–98; L. L. Heston and J. Shields, "Homosexuality in Twins," *Archives of General Psychiatry* 18 (1968): 149–60.

40. See, for instance, G. Klintworth, "A Pair of Male Monozygotic Twins Discordant for Homosexuality," *Journal of Nervous and Mental Disorders* 135 (1962): 113–25.

41. Sigmund Freud, *Three Essays on the Theory of Sexuality* (1905), in *Collected Works of Freud*, ed. J. Stachey, 7 vols. (London: Hogarth, 1953).

42. See especially Weinrich, "Strategy." This dissertation is essential reading for anyone interested in human sociobiology.

43. Some clarification is necessary here. A man who puts on a bra and panties because it "turns him on" is a transvestite. Most transvestities are as heterosexual, if not more, than conventional heterosexuals. A cross dresser aims to excite members of his/her own sex. A male prostitute in "drag" is a cross-dresser.

44. Weinrich, "Strategy," p. 170.

45. Ibid, p. 171.

46. Ibid.

47. Ibid, p. 173.

48. Ibid.

49. Ibid.

50. Ibid, p. 129.
51. Ibid, pp. 203–5.
52. Ibid, p. 175.
53. Ibid.
54. Ibid, p. 176.

Bioethics and the Human Prospect

VAN RENSSELAER POTTER

University of Wisconsin

People of good will need to enlarge their concerns beyond the issues in medical bioethics that many people identify as the subject matter for the new discipline of bioethics. There is a backlash against medical science and against science and technology in general. The incidence of malpractice suits is at an all-time high, and physicians complain that insurance costs have become prohibitive. Suits at the level of one or two million dollars for a damaged or lost life have become commonplace. The monetary value of a human life is incalculable, but these monetary judgments form the backdrop against which the current interest in individual human rights must be viewed. Issues of abortion, contraception, death with dignity, euthanasia, and the final issue of the right to choose the time of death are all subsumed in bioethics. For this we are indebted to the tremendous upsurge in scholarly activity in this area at the Institute at Hastings and at the Center for Bioethics at Georgetown University. Without in any way detracting from these important centers, I want to emphasize that bioethics covers a broader subject than these efforts suggest. Already we need an adjective to specify what kind of bioethics is to be discussed. The above centers are mainly concerned with medical bioethics, which is essentially medical ethics in an age in which ethical decisions are difficult because of the options afforded by medical technology. In the old days the first rule in medical ethics was to do nothing unless absolutely sure that doing something would not make the patient worse. This was the rule of *primum non nocere*. Today, medical doctors are pushed by patients and relatives "to do something." So Hastings and Georgetown are performing a service by illuminating the ethical dilemmas created by the availability of options.

Meanwhile, another branch of bioethics has developed, which may be referred to as bioethics in the Wisconsin tradition, or environmental bioethics. I feel justified in speaking of the Wisconsin tradition not only because I am of that school but also because of the heritage that has come to me through John Muir and Aldo Leopold, who are nationally known to conservationists. John Muir spent four years at the University of Wisconsin and later promoted the idea of national forests. Aldo Leopold, a Wisconsin professor, died fighting his neighbor's grassfire in 1948, but his book, *A Sand County Almanac,*[1] published posthumously in 1949, is widely known. At the Institute for Environmental Studies at the University of Wisconsin, courses are now being offered in environmental bioethics, and it is hoped that this effort will lead to further education in this field, which owes so much to Aldo Leopold.

Just as medical bioethics is concerned with the life and death of particular individuals, environmental bioethics is concerned with the life and possible death of human society—that is to say, the human prospect. The phrase—the human prospect—has a distinguished past and a recent history. It was used by a great pioneer in environmental bioethics, Lewis Mumford, although he never employed the term *bioethics*. His book, entitled *The Human Prospect,* was published in 1955.[2] Environmental bioethics is about survival, not of individuals, but of humankind. When we speak of the human prospect, we think of the future; we think of the probabilities of human survival in acceptable form and what chance we have to affect the outcome. Mumford's *The Human Prospect* included "Notes for a New Age" and an essay entitled "Program for Survival," which was taken from Mumford's *Values for Survival,* published in 1946. Mumford was indeed as much a prophet as Leopold for the coming age of environmental bioethics. *The Human Prospect* is a handbook of philosophy for the future: "The aim is not more goods for more people to buy, but more opportunities for them to live: hence only such increases in goods as are instrumental to 'the best life possible' " (p. 249).

At present we need to integrate the views of those writers who have expressed concern about the longterm human prospect. Cutting across all of the individual points of view is the central problem of how political systems can best cope with human nature in the long run. Later in this essay I propose the basic bioethic as the only possible solution I can visualize. Few authors have dealt with the problem more cogently than Robert Heilbroner in his 1974 book entitled *An Inquiry into the Human Prospect,* which opens with the following:

> There is a question in the air, more sensed than seen, like the invisible approach of a distant storm, a question that I would hesitate to ask aloud did I not believe it existed unvoiced in the minds of many: "Is there hope for man?"
>
> In another era such a question might have raised thoughts of man's ultimate salvation or damnation. But today the brooding doubts that it arouses have to do with life on earth, now, and in the relatively few generations that constitute the limit of our capacity to imagine the future. For the question asks whether we can imagine that future other than as a continuation of the darkness, cruelty, and disorder of the past; worse, whether we do not foresee in the human prospect a deterioration of things, even an impending catastrophe of fearful dimensions.[3]

Heilbroner speaks of a civilizational malaise that reflects the inability of a civilization directed toward material improvements (higher incomes, better diets, miracles of medicine, triumphs of applied physics and chemistry) to satisfy the human spirit. Heilbroner notes the possibility that humanity may react to the approach of environmental collapse by indulging in a vast fling while it is still possible. Perhaps this explains the upsurge in the purchase of large automobiles just after the first Arab oil embargo crisis had passed.

Another book concerned with the human prospect is by Erik Eckholm of Worldwatch Institute. This book is intended to be a realistic survey of food prospects, and it is entitled *Losing Ground.*[4] The grim realities are seen in every sector, whether in terms of world fishing, mountain communities, tropical agriculture, or the export-import relationship between North America and the rest of the world. The increasing human population seems to be on a collision course with the downward spiral of decreasing efficiency in global food production. The urgent need for bringing these opposing trends into balance poses moral problems, not just economic ones, and the call is for accelerating the development of environmental bioethics. We must attempt to develop a rational, moral approach to the balancing of the needs and aspirations of present generations against the needs and aspirations of future generations, recognizing that inappropriate present decisions can foreclose the very possibility of existence for future generations. What I am emphasizing is that medical bioethics needs to operate in the perspective of environmental bioethics. The former deals with individuals now; the latter deals with the survival of society, which is necessary for a decent life for individuals in the future.

THE MEANING OF SURVIVAL

The problem posed for environmental bioethics by a consideration of the human prospect is the question of survival. In the past it was always assumed, as noted by Darwin, that the wide dispersion of the human species guaranteed survival against catastrophes that were assumed to be localized. Later, with atomic and nuclear explosions, worldwide devastation could be imagined. Still later, worldwide damage by nuclear proliferation; resource depletion; disseminated manmade pollution; invasion by insects, other pests, and parasites; and breakdown in health facilities could be envisioned on a wide scale. The present situation is that the preservation or destruction of the earth's ecosystem and its people is clearly in the hands of the human species. The responsibility is ours. By ours I mean the few people who have the intelligence to see the problems and the luxury to contemplate them. I will note here that responsibility is part of the basic bioethic.

The titles of books on survival are suggestive: Mumford's *Values of Survival,* Vogt's *Road to Survival,* Neutra's *Design for Survival,* Meeker's *The Comedy of Survival,* and Callahan's *The Tyranny of Survival.* These titles involve nouns: values, road, design, comedy, and tyranny. I should like to discuss five different kinds of survival in terms of five qualifying adjectives: *mere, miserable, idealistic, irresponsible,* and *acceptable.*

Mere survival is the kind of existence that is mentioned among the questions I get routinely when advocating bioethics as the science of survival. Are we interested only in mere survival? The answer is no. We are also concerned with human values, but even today in many communities, mere survival would be better than what people have, which is my second category, *miserable survival.* Large segments of the world population live today with malnutrition, parasitic infection, preventable disease, and high rates of infant mortality. Even in our own society, mental breakdown, advanced senility, alcoholism, and drug addiction threaten many. It is impossible to specify ideal survival, but it is possible to seek a third category, *idealistic survival,* as a goal that would eliminate miserable survival and also would seek to avoid my fourth category, which is *irresponsible survival.* It is irresponsible for a society to place its highest value on material gadgetry and on rates of energy consumption that far exceed the amounts needed. These conclusions lead to the fifth category, which I call *acceptable survival.*

We cannot agree today on what would be universally acceptable, but, adhering to the basic bioethic, we can agree on guidelines that might be helpful. I can state without reservation that the majority of the U.S. population is now engaged in irresponsible survival without regard for future descendants or our present global neighbors. The reasons are not malevolent but rather stem from the cultural heritage of the majority. As Heilbroner has pointed out, any kind of a cultural turnaround is difficult to imagine, although Mumford has been calling for one for over forty years. With a moderate amount of research we could make a list of items that could be deleted from our options without producing malnutrition, disease, or any lack of outlet for creative or other pleasurable endeavor. I would offer, for example, skis and snowshoes or even hiking boots as substitutes for snowmobiles. Canoes and sailboats could substitute for motorboats. In the health field, pure water could replace artificially sweetened cola drinks; walking could replace some transportation needs; and healthful food could be provided at a fraction of its present cost. More serious discussions could lead to energy independence within three years and even further savings in the future. The emphasis here is that while irresponsible survival is the rule at present, an acceptable survival is not too difficult to imagine. What is difficult to contemplate is any sort of a turnaround in our national ethos unless it is precipitated by a major catastrophe.

In a booklet entitled "Human Values on the Spaceship Earth," published in 1966 by the National Council of the Churches of Christ (U.S.A.), the authors discussed many aspects of what I call acceptable survival and stressed two conclusions: (1) "radical changes in society demand courageous and imaginative changes in theology and ethics" and (2) "the common good takes precedence over the self-interest of individuals or any partisan group in the community." Whether these ideas can be applied globally is open to question, but at least they speak out against irresponsible survival. What is needed for acceptable survival is a set of bioethical axioms or value judgments that can first be agreed upon and second used as a basis for research and further decisions. As we contemplate the spaceship Earth as seen from outer space, we should realize that there are no lifeboats in case of failure and no opportunity to launch another ship. We have to make it on this one or none at all.

AXIOMS FOR ENVIRONMENTAL BIOETHICS

An axiom cannot be proved; it can only be accepted, rejected, or modified on the basis of considerable dialogue. I now propose an overall axiom for environmental bioethics:

1. Survival of the human species in acceptable form is desirable. This axiom cannot be discussed at length, but it is taken as given that human survival over long periods comparable to man's known past cannot be assumed. It is further recognized that a definition of acceptable survival requires much study and research. It is emphasized that such discussion and research are not now taking place to any significant extent.

Under this major axiom are three additional axioms that have been proposed by Ronald Green,[5] a former student of John Rawls, who is well known for his book *A Theory of Justice*. Green's axioms are:

2. We are bound by ties of justice to real future persons.
3. The lives of future persons ideally ought to be "better" than our own and certainly no worse.
4. Sacrifices on behalf of the future must be distributed equitably in the present with special regard for those least advantaged.

The first four axioms must be viewed in the perspective of a fifth axiom:

5. Survival of the human species in acceptable form demands adherence, in general, to the Leopold Imperative: "A thing is right when it tends to preserve the integrity, stability, and beauty of the biotic community. It is wrong when it tends to do otherwise."

What we must now undertake is a realistic appraisal of the implications and qualifications of the final two axioms. The problem is whether a viable balance of distributive justice (Rawls's term) can be achieved among (1) future generations, (2) presently affluent populations, and (3) presently miserable populations, using a healthy ecosystem as an unwavering standard. After all, if the ecosystem breaks down, none of the three competing populations in the distributive dilemma can survive. This leads us back to the problem of developing environmental bioethics.

ORIGINS OF ENVIRONMENTAL BIOETHICS

It is appropriate to look for a moment at one of the early pronouncements on environmental bioethics. In a series of papers M. Torchio emphasized the traditions of the Benedictine monasteries as among the earliest evidence of explicit bioethical concerns.[6] Thus, he cited an important work, "On the Conservation of Pine Forests" by the abbot of the Benedictine Congregation of Vallombrosa in 1804:

> . . . no one who plants a fir-tree can hope to fell it when it is fully grown, no matter how youthful the person is. In spite of this the most sacred obligation is to replant and husband these pine forests. If we sweat for the benefit of posterity, we should not complain as we reap the results of the efforts of our forefathers. . . . Not one of our forebears survives now nor shall we do when those who follow on cut down the trees that we planted for them.

I am not aware of any evidence that this Benedictine contribution influenced the later thinking of Theodore Roosevelt, Gifford Pinchot, John Muir, Henry Thoreau, or other American conservationists, but it is worth mentioning that there is a clear line of evolving environmental bioethics that may be referred to as the Wisconsin tradition, which runs, as mentioned before, from John Muir to Aldo Leopold and more recently to an explicit series of beliefs and commitments that are part of a bioethical creed and to the present discussion.[7]

ENVIRONMENTAL VALUES: INTRINSIC OR SECONDARY?

Holmes Rolston has discussed the contributions of Aldo Leopold and others in terms of the basic question of whether the natural environment should be preserved because of an intrinsic worth, or whether the environment should be valued because of its contribution to the present and future welfare of the human species: are environmental values intrinsic and primary, or are they merely a matter of social expediency, that is, secondary?[8] Rolston has argued that "to say that the balance of nature is a ground for human values is not to draw any ethics from ecology, as may first appear, but only to recognize the necessary medium of ethical activity."[9] An environmental ethic based on intrinsic value of the ecosystem does not mean that there is an intrinsic ethic in the ecosystem since ethics requires a conscious self-awareness, other-awareness, and death-awareness presently ascribed only to human beings able to communicate with each other. The ecosystem has ground rules and boundary conditions from which biologists can discern and draw inferences, but it seems inappropriate to speak of an intrinsic ethic in the ecosystem. What deserves to be emphasized is the basis for ascribing value to the ecosystem and the need for an environmental bioethic that can affect cultural development.

Rolston has credited Leopold with the clearest affirmation of the intrinsic ethical lesson for man within the ecosystem. This is expressed in the statement I have referred to as the Leopold Imperative. From this Rolston has found "homeostasis a key to all values. The precondition of values, if you will—but one which for all that, informs and shapes (man's) other values by making them relational, corporate, environmental." Such a view is morally prescriptive for man: ". . . given options within parameters of necessary obedience, he morally ought to promote (environmental) homeostasis."[10]

TOWARD ENVIRONMENTAL BIOETHICS AS A DISCIPLINE

Rolston's views and his interpretation of Leopold's ethic are completely in accord with my own position as expressed in my *Bioethics, Bridge to the Future,* which was dedicated to the memory of Aldo Leopold, "who anticipated the extension of ethics to Bioethics." In this book I stated that ". . . ethics implies action according to moral standards. What we must now face up to is the fact that human ethics cannot be separated from a realistic understanding of ecology in the broadest sense. Ethical values cannot be separated from biological facts. . . . Survival of the total ecosystem is the test of the value system" (pp. vii–viii). In my dedication to *Bioethics, Bridge to the Future* I quoted from Aldo Leopold's *A Sand County Almanac* in much the same spirit: "An ethic may be regarded as a mode of guidance for meeting ecological situations so new or intricate, or involving such deferred reactions that the path of social expediency is not discernible to the average individual" (*Sand County Almanac,* p. 203). In relating ethics to action I really mean activity or behavior, since I have explained (*Bioethics,* p. 185) that Kant had observed that wisdom could be looked upon as an action policy for doing or letting be.

Since Leopold's time, the further exposition of environmental dilemmas has been taken up in many publications by Garrett Hardin. Leopold was searching for a morality of land use that would escape economic expediency as distinct from social expediency. He was trying to advance the ethical frontier from the merely interpersonal to the region of man in transaction with his environment.[11] Similarly, Hardin has introduced the concept of environmental disaster through expanding population plus shortsighted, self-interested, economic exploitation of the public domain.[12] His conclusion puts human survival on an ethical basis: "The population problem has no technical solution: it requires a fundamental extension in morality." Hardin's prescription is "mutual coercion, mutually agreed upon," a concept to which we will return later. Meanwhile, in a reply to Hardin, Beryl Crowe has come to the sobering conclusion that "major problems have neither technical nor political solutions: extensions in morality are not likely."[13]

In an attempt to visualize what might be called the "tragedy of the commons averted," I have generated a sequence appropriate to the present analysis:

1. Environmental damage becomes visible to Leopold's "average individual"; moral indignation is aroused.
2. Knowledge of the problems and their time scales in "ecological situations so new or intricate, or involving such deferred reactions" (Leopold) evolves into a new discipline: environmental bioethics.
3. Moral indignation seeks preventive and creative countermeasures.
4. Moral pressure plus factual information generates bioethical guidelines.
5. Moral pressure converts bioethical guidelines into legal sanctions; i.e., "moral coercion mutually agreed upon" (Hardin).

This scenario cannot be given a timetable except to say that the march of events is rapidly outpacing developments in environmental bioethics and the conversion to and implementation of laws derived therefrom.

In moving toward the development of an environmental bioethic, I have attempted to state my conception of ethic, which is the broader term for a medical bioethic or an environmental bioethic: *an ethic is a set of culturally accepted beliefs and guidelines for decisions affecting the course of human activity, with idealistic goals in mind, usually involving the adjustment of competing claims without resorting to the use of coercion.*

In considering this definition, we may note that the world in general and the United States in particular is not culturally homogeneous, a point strongly emphasized by Crowe when he doubted the occurrence of "extensions in morality." There is, however, probably no culture that places a premium on ill health, malnutrition, parasitic infection, or infant mortality per se. If these can be shown to be the outcome of political systems and laws that fail to recognize the minimal requirements of a healthy ecosystem, leadership may develop that will avert the "tragedy of the commons."

To paraphrase Rolston, environmental bioethics evolves rather straightforwardly from classical ethical queries that are now advised of certain ecological boundaries. The ultimate science of environmental bioethics

> may well herald limits to growth; it challenges certain presumptions about rising standards of living, capitalism, progress, development, and so on; convictions that, though deeply entrenched

> parameters of human value, are issues of what is, can, or will be the case, not of what ought to be. This realization of limits . . . can hardly be said to reform our ethical roots, for the reason that its scope remains (when optimistic) a maximizing of human values or (when pessimistic) human survival.[14]

Rolston has concluded that

> much of the search for an ecological morality will, perhaps in necessary pragmatism, remain secondary, "conservative," where the ground is better charted, and where we mix ethics, science, and human interests under our logical control. But we judge the ethical frontier to be beyond a primary revaluing where, in ethical creativity, conscience must evolve. The topography is largely uncharted; to cross it will require the daring, and caution, of a community of scientists and ethicists who can together map both the ecosystem and the ethical grammar appropriate for it.[15]

THE BASIC BIOETHIC

In the development of a community of scientists and ethicists who can learn from each other and develop a new discipline, I can suggest nothing more basic than the "bioethic of humility with responsibility."[16] Responsibility implies competence, and humility implies a willingness to admit shortcomings and inadequacies of single-purpose planning and single-discipline discourse. Humility implies a willingness to listen to people from other disciplines and other walks of life. Certainly the combined virtues of humility, responsibility, and competence are necessary if we are to have individuals who are both scientists and ethicists.

Stephen Tonsor has called for an end to the traditional separation between science and ethics.[17] Kluckhohn had earlier commented on the failure of the scientific enterprise to develop "a system of general ideas and values that would give meaning to human life in the mid-twentieth century," and he blamed the failure on the belief by individual scientists that ethics was the property of the church and outside their responsibility.[18] Now Tonsor, discussing the articulation of revolt and despair by writers and artists,[19] has argued for a new emphasis on the ethical dimension in higher education:

> If we are to teach, to educate, we must start where men are now. . . . The godly and the godless alike are troubled and confused by a world in which moral consensus has all but disappeared but in which men must continue to act to their future woe or weal. Decisions must be made, choices acted on, preferences voiced. We are able to suspend belief but we are unable to suspend action. The fundamental debates of this time are ethical debates. . . . If we are to act ecumenically, let us begin not with Theology but with ethics. . . . Let the moral debate begin not with questions about the existence of God or the immortality of the soul but with a discussion of the nature of man and the avenues through which men can fulfill their natural existences. The realm of grace will disclose itself in due time and the ultimate questions of meaning will intrude themselves. I do not pretend that this "naturalistic" ethic will save men's souls but it will enable them to live together in civil society and will put them in a position to ask far more searching and meaningful questions. . . . If we cannot agree on how we should act there is little hope that we shall agree on what we are to believe.[20]

As a first step in relating belief to action, I have previously proposed six statements of belief and commitment for action in a bioethical creed, which I need not reiterate here.[21] Building on the bioethical creed, I now propose six goals for environmental bioethics that are prescriptive responses to the five axioms I mentioned earlier:

1. Decreased world population;
2. Increased food self-sufficiency;
3. Increased public health measures;
4. Decreased energy and resource consumption relative to U.S. average;
5. Priority for essential technology;
6. Definition of acceptable and responsible survival.

The relevance of these goals is predicated on an overview of the human prospect as may be visualized in the chart shown in fig. 1. In this chart I emphasize the need for the application of the basic bioethic of humility, responsibility, and competence to the evolution of a body of precepts that may be categorized as Evolutionary Bioethics, recalling the contributions of Muir, Leopold, Hardin, Crowe, Green, Rolston, and Tonsor, as described here.[22] This chart stresses that future generations will be consigned to an acceptable survival or to a miserable sur-

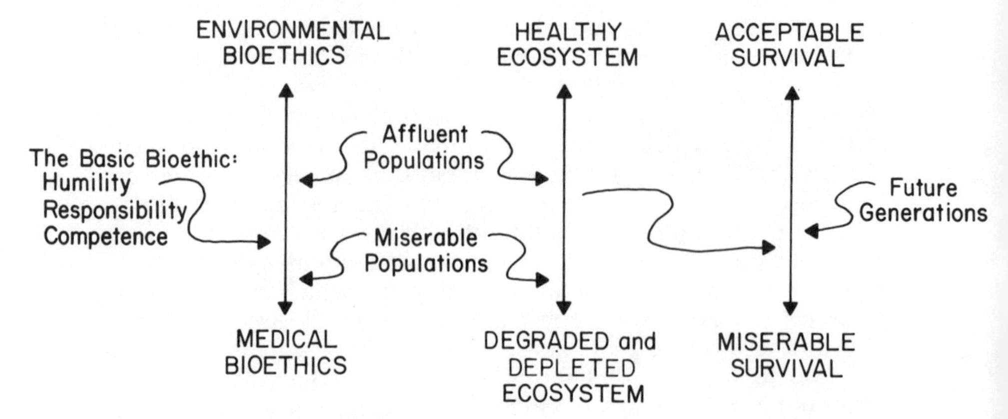

FIG. 1. The human prospect seen as dependent upon the maintenance of a healthy ecosystem. The vertical arrows represent competing options. The horizontal arrows represent factors affecting the balance between the options. A healthy ecosystem is essential for survival of future generations but is under attack from both affluent and miserable populations. If medical bioethics concentrates on death control without achieving adequate birth control, the result can lead to an expansion of miserable populations, to a degraded and depleted ecosystem, and to future populations condemned to a miserable survival. Environmental bioethics is proposed as a multidisciplinary approach for individuals concerned with global problems.

vival depending on whether present generations maintain a healthy ecosystem or produce a degraded and depleted ecosystem, and it further indicates that the forces influencing the balance are not solely the result of actions by either the affluent Western populations or the miserable masses of people in the underdeveloped parts of the world. Both contribute to the degradation and depletion of the ecosystem and will continue to do so unless a much wider acceptance of the basic bioethic can lead to an evolving set of guidelines, laws, and actions that are based on the overall concepts of environmental bioethics.

NOTES

1. *A Sand County Almanac* (New York: Oxford University Press, 1949, 1953, 1966).
2. *The Human Prospect* (Boston: Beacon Press, 1955).
3. *An Inquiry into the Human Prospect* (New York: W. W. Norton, 1974), p. 13.
4. *Losing Ground, Environmental Stress and World Prospects* (New York: W. W. Norton, 1976).

5. Ronald Green, "Intergenerational Distributive Justice and Environmental Responsibility," *BioScience* 27 (1977): 260–65.

6. M. Torchio, and R. C. Torchio, "Studi ed uso razionale della Natura nei Benedettini italiani dell'evo moderno," *Natura* (Milano) 63 (1972): 205–55; M. Torchio, "Rapporti unomo-Natura secondo le principali metafisiche orientali, loro implicazioni bioetiche ed ecologiche," *Natura* (Milano) 64 (1973): 101–32; M. Torchio "Bioethics: A Bridge to Survival" (1975, unpublished MS).

7. See my *Bioethics, Bridge to the Future* (Englewood Cliffs, N.J.: Prentice-Hall, 1971).

8. See Holmes Rolston, "Philosophical Aspects of the Environment," in *Environment and Colorado: A Handbook*, ed. Phillip O. Foss (Fort Collins, Col.: Environmental Resources, Colorado State University, 1974); "Is There an Ecological Ethic?" *Ethics* 85 (1975): 93–109.

9. Rolston, "Is There an Ecological Ethic?", p. 98.

10. Ibid., p. 99.

11. Rolston, "Is There an Ecological Ethic?", p. 99.

12. Garrett Hardin, "The Tragedy of the Commons," *Science* 162 (1968): 1243–48.

13. Beryl Crowe, "The Tragedy of the Commons Revisited," *Science* 166 (1969): 1103–7.

14. Rolston, "Is there an Ecological Ethic?," p. 98.

15. Ibid., p. 109.

16. See my "Humility with Responsibility, the Basic Bioethic," *Wisconsin Academy Reviews* 21 (1975): 18–20; "Humility with Responsibility—a Bioethic for Oncologists: Presidential Address," *Cancer Research* 35 (1975): 2297–306.

17. Stephen Tonsor, "Why John Newman Was Wrong: The Connection Between Moral and Intellectual Virtue in Higher Education" (Paper delivered at Symposium at Bellarmine College, Louisville, Ky., January 23, 1974).

18. C. Kluckhohn, "The Scientific Study of Values and Contemporary Civilization," *Proceedings of the American Philosophical Society* 120 (1959): 468–76.

19. Stephen Tonsor, "The Iconography of Disorder: The Ruined Garden and the Devastated City," *Modern Age* 17 (1973): 358–67.

20. Tonsor; "Why John Newman Was Wrong."

21. See my "Bioethics for Whom?," *Annals of New York Academy of Science* 196 (1972): 200–205 (table 1).

22. Portions of this essay are reproduced from a short introduction to a special section of *BioScience* for April 1977, with permission. See V. R. Potter, "Evolving Ethical Concepts," *BioScience* 27 (1977): 251–53. The present essay is adapted from the unpublished Keynote Lecture, "Bioethics and the Future of the Human Enterprise," at a Symposium at the College of Mount St. Joseph-on-the-Ohio on July 11, 1976.

Patients in Particular: Three Cases in Clinical Management

W. J. COGGINS

University of Alabama College of Community Health Services

and
PETER GRAHAM

Virginia Polytechnic Institute and State University

Writing about the intellectual basis of family practice, G. Gale Stephens suggests that the quintessential skill and crucial feature characterizing the specialty is patient management.[1] What distinguishes the family physician is not that he takes care of all or even several members of a family but that he thinks of his patient as a person in a family, endeavors to understand the particulars of this situation, and plans a course of treatment in light of the insights he gains. Thus the family physician is the sort of doctor Philip Tumulty describes at the beginning of *The Effective Clinician,* "one whose prime function is to manage a sick person with the purpose of alleviating most effectively the total impact of illness upon that person."[2] The family physician, along with other practitioners mainly concerned with patient care, acts on a small stage and plays to a limited audience. No priestly intermediary, he does not merely transmit or administer remedies but also participates actively in the healing process. Understanding medical problems in context, striving to perceive the genetic, psychological, social, cultural, economic, and environmental particulars that impinge on the patient and modify his illness, the doctor equips himself to treat a person, not a complaint.

Accurate diagnosis is not the most crucial part of the clinician's job. His paramount task is to help the sufferer, whether he can satisfactorily identify a medical problem or not.[3] There are instances, however, when his medical authority will not suffice to implement the appropriate therapy. Inadequate communication between doctor and patient or unacknowledged disparities between what the two parties understand the problem to be can hinder treatment. In such circumstances the physician, exercising his powers of imagination and empathy, should become a bridge-builder. He should endeavor to discover the dimensions of the problem as it exists in the mind of his patient and, by establishing a common frame of reference, should bring the patient to a point at which effective treatment will be possible.[4] The case of "Uncle Charlie" shows how such a shared frame of reference can be constructed.

Uncle Charlie was a sixty-year-old mullet fisherman who was recognized in the community as a harmless eccentric. He lived alone in a shack at the northernmost tip of an island where everyone else lived at the south end. Since other shacks were available, his choice appeared to me to be more than a random selection. His behavior when I would see him on the streets did not seem particularly avuncular, and I was puzzled by the title until I realized that this was the community's way of saying that in being no one's uncle, Uncle Charlie became everyone's.

He came to my office one day complaining of an eye problem and went on to explain that he had fish scales coming out of his eyes. He said that in his many years of catching, handling, and cleaning fish he had absorbed thousands of fish scales into his system and now they were coming out. His eyes were very red and irritated. Every two or three minutes during our interview he would put his fingers in his eyes and extract small amounts of matter. These he showed me, explaining that they were fish scales. I agreed that there was something there and that he did indeed have a problem. I learned that he read the Bible regularly and wondered, but did not ask, if the statement, "If thine eye offends thee, pluck it out," had any particular meaning to him. The frequency and vigor with which he picked at his eyes during the interview alarmed me. I had a macabre fantasy of his doing just that while digging for the offending fish scales.

My examination showed nothing except for irritation of his eyes and a mild ectropion, but he was also in early congestive heart failure. I wanted to treat his heart failure because he worked hard and was often out in his boat alone. I prescribed digitalis and gave him some harmless drops for his eyes. When he returned a week later, his eyes were no better, and he had disdained to take his heart pills. . . .

At his second meeting with Uncle Charlie, the doctor inferred that his uncooperative patient had resisted the prescribed treatment because of an unreconciled difference in their respective perceptions of the complaint. Uncle Charlie had come to be treated for something other than what the doctor had found to be his major somatic problem. Uncle Charlie's psychological state further complicated the picture: he was, mentally as well as geographically, out of touch with the world. The physician's first task, then, was to determine in what ways his diagnosis and Uncle Charlie's were at odds. Armed with this knowledge, he would then translate his course of treatment into terms that Uncle Charlie could find acceptable. The chart below traces the identification and solution of this tactical problem:

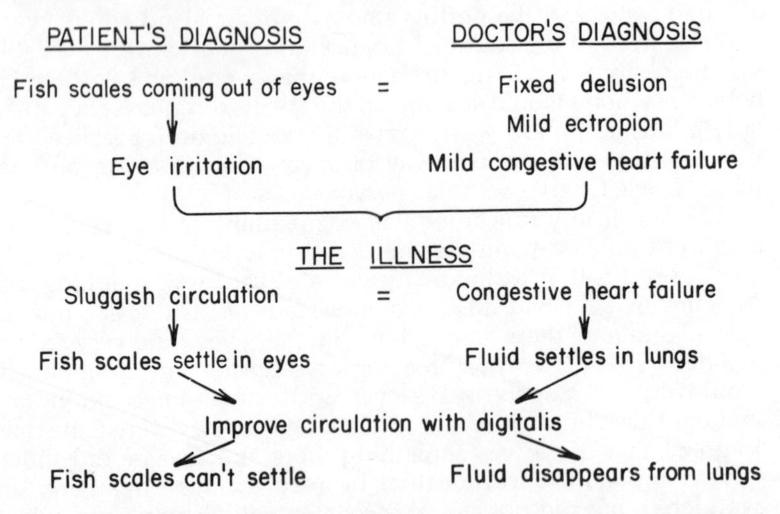

Uncle Charlie had come on account of—and demanded to be treated for—fish scales. From the physician's standpoint, of course, this complaint was a side issue, a neurotic misconception that motivated a pattern of behavior (rubbing and picking at the eyes) that in turn heightened a minor physiological problem. What warranted treatment was the fisherman's heart failure. But how would the doctor enlist Uncle Charlie's active compliance, without which therapy could not succeed?

As it turned out, the most expedient way to reconcile the patient's convictions with the medical diagnosis was to present the main somatic difficulty (mild congestive heart failure) in such a way that Uncle Charlie would perceive it as *causally* linked with the problem of fish scales. "Sluggish circulation," which in fact did allow fluid to build up in Uncle Charlie's lungs, could be presented as the culprit that enabled the fish scales to settle in his eyes. Digitalis, Uncle Charlie was told, would improve his circulation; hence the fish scales would be unable to settle. This explanation sufficed to enlist the patient's support. Uncle Charlie took the digitalis. His heart condition improved, and having been convinced that the fish scales were no longer obtruding themselves, he ceased to irritate his eyes. The doctor's plan of action had satisfactorily resolved the problems identified by both parties.

Viewed superficially, such willingness to accommodate medical facts to Uncle Charlie's delusions might seem to violate the "patient's right to know." But, given Uncle Charlie's intellectual and social isolation, educating him about his condition would have been virtually impossible as well as unnecessary. Uncle Charlie's reclusive habits and reputation for eccentricity made it unlikely that his "fish scales" delusion would encounter public opposition. Furthermore, if the physician had tried and failed to press his own interpretation of the case, to enlighten Uncle Charlie on the subjects of cardiac failure, ectropion, and his fixed delusion, he would have lost his credibility and with it his chance to assist the patient.

Perhaps the crucial component in the successful *modus operandi* for treating Uncle Charlie was the doctor's awareness that his patient's heart condition, inextricably allied with his minor physical problems, mental quirks, and social circumstances, could not be remedied in isolation from Uncle Charlie's view of reality. The doctor understood that as clinical manager he was treating an eccentric fisherman, not a mere case of congestive heart failure. In order to care effectively for this particular patient, the doctor made the necessary efforts to meet him on his own terms. Acquiescing in the matter of the fish scales, the physician sacrificed medical explanations so that treatment might carry the day. His chosen course of action involved neither knuckling under nor condescending to Uncle

Charlie. Instead, by empathetically constructing a shared frame of reference, he drew the patient onto ground from which the two could work as a team against Uncle Charlie's illness, whatever the name.

Perceptual problems such as those that impeded treatment of Uncle Charlie's complaint are not the only uncertainties the clinician encounters. In the following case of an otherwise healthy man with a highly malignant cancer of the skin, diagnosis and communication proved simple. The critical question here was one of patient management. Given the general character of the disease and the specific circumstances of the patient, the doctor had to decide which of two risk-fraught alternatives would prove less hazardous.

> A fifty-year-old traveling salesman complained of a large, growing mole on his back. I performed an excision biopsy. The surgical pathologist's report identified the excised tissue as an intact malignant melanoma. I referred my patient to a highly regarded surgeon, who advised radical neck and axillary dissection as soon as possible. This operation, because it would mutilate parts of the arm and the chest wall, would carry with it morbidity secondary to the surgical procedure itself.
>
> I realized that my patient's work required him to carry heavy cases of samples in and out of business offices all day long and that he had experienced a period of unemployment several years earlier when the store where he had long been a clerk had failed. As a salesman the patient had worked hard to build up his route to the point where he could support his family of five comfortably if he worked twelve to fourteen hours a day. He had no disability insurance. His wife had no vocational skills.
>
> Having reviewed the literature on melanoma, I consulted by telephone with a second surgeon, who suggested that the radical neck and axillary dissection, still an experimental procedure, was not imperative. I then advised the patient against any further surgery. The patient complied with considerable relief and returned to work. He retired some fifteen years later and died at age seventy of unrelated cause.

Despite its clear-cut diagnosis, the salesman's case remained ambiguous for several reasons. Although the melanoma had been removed in its entirety, cancer cells can metastasize through the bloodstream and after a time reappear elsewhere. The radical neck and axillary dissection might or might not have reduced the possibility of recurrence. Coping with the operation and its consequences might have proved as dangerous to the patient as was the disease itself. The removal of chest and arm tissue would have prevented the salesman from returning to his arduous job. Unable to rely on other sources of income, he probably would have had to start anew for a third time—a demoralizing prospect for a middle-aged convalescent. In deciding not to recommend further treatment, the doctor gambled that the mental stress attendant on the operation outweighed the possible return of the disease: "waiting out" the situation seemed, of two uncertainties, the one this particular patient could best face. In this instance, the gamble paid off, though in withholding medical action the doctor took upon himself some of the anxiety from which he had freed his patient.

The clinician's main job is to help his patients get well, but his responsibilities do not end when the chances for recovery run out. His guidance and support can help the patient and his family to confront imminent death. In the following narrative of terminal illness, the family physician permitted his patient to seek treatments that he did not sanction. Nurturing the family's emotional adjustment to the coming bereavement, the clinical manager forbore pressing his medical views.

> During a routine physical examination, I found that a thirteen-year-old boy had an asymptomatic lump in his lower back. I immediately referred the patient to an orthopedic surgeon, who performed an open biopsy that revealed cancer of the bony spine. I then sent the boy to New York for radiation therapy. The treatment caused no regression in the tumor. Informed by the New York specialist that nothing further could be done, the boy's parents brought him home to await death.
>
> Soon after their return, the family asked me to consent to their trying treatment at a naturopathic hospital in Denver, Colorado. The cost would be $10,000, but the family had a rich patron, the father's employer. A telephone call to the naturopathic hospital satisfied me that the treatment, a regimen of herbal remedies and vegetarian diet, would be harmless, and I gave my consent. After two weeks in Denver, the patient and his family returned home by way of an Oral Roberts "faith healing" session in Kansas City. The patient lived only two months longer, but the anxiety, depression, and despair the family had felt on their return from radiation therapy had vanished. All bases had been touched.

Here the physician had either to refuse a suffering family the support they required or to acquiesce as they resorted to what some of his colleagues might term "sectarian methods" and others might call "quackery." Several factors combined to permit his compliance with the family's wishes. The doctor understood that the unconventional treatments would not harm the patient or cripple the family's finances. More important, he saw that for peace of mind these particular people needed to try all alternatives, but, because they recognized that the odds against a miracle cure were high, also needed to know that their family doctor would stand by them if all else failed. Once satisfied that they had done everything they could, the family faced the prospect of death with the equanimity they had hitherto lacked. The doctor's empathy, though it could not save the patient, helped preserve the family's emotional health.

Different as they are, these three case studies all suggest a final point: the family physician may be a generalist, but generalizations have limited use in his practice. Dr. Peter Medawar has defended scientific reductionism with a phrase borrowed from William Blake. Medical research, Medawar writes, is obliged "to do good in minute particulars."[5] The clinician too works in a microcosm. However sophisticated his theoretical background, however subtle his diagnostic skills, he uses his arts in small, specific engagements. He does not offer a paradigm of health but mends, patches, and if need be manipulates the individuals under his care, so that each may regain his own self-defined state of wellness. The doctor is doomed and privileged to do good in minute particulars, one patient at a time.

NOTES

1. G. Gayle Stephens, "The Intellectual Basis of Family Practice," *Journal of Family Practice* 2 (1975): 423–28.
2. Philip A. Tumulty, *The Effective Clinician* (Philadelphia: W. B. Saunders, 1973), p. 1.
3. Stephens, "The Intellectual Basis."
4. Michael Balint, *The Doctor, His Patient, and the Illness* (New York: International Universities Press, 1972).
5. Peter B. Medawar, "Some Follies of Prediction," *Hospital Practice* 10 (1975): 73–74.

Health, Art, and Drama: Underutilized Resources for Improved Quality of Life

DENNIS CARLSON

Johns Hopkins School of Hygiene and Public Health

> The vitality and energies of the imagination do not operate at will; they are fountains not machinery.
>
> D. G. James, *Skepticism and Poetry*

Health requires more than modern medicine currently has to offer.[1] The well-being implied in the ideal of "health" necessitates a satisfying balance of physical, psychological, and spiritual processes that goes beyond the absence, removal, or alleviation of disease.[2] Many medical scientists and physicians would concur with this widely accepted meaning of health but still would insist that at the present time their chief focus must remain on the dynamics of illness. Moreover, their methods and assumptions focus on the study of problems that can be objectively observed and systematically quantified.[3] No one would deny the enormous benefits that have been achieved by this approach. Nevertheless, many people in industrialized societies would agree with the title of a recent issue of *Daedalus* that we are "Doing Better and Feeling Worse."[4] Other pressures, such as the rising cost of hospital services and the problem of providing equitable accessibility, contribute to the widespread belief that the treatment and prevention of disease are insufficient. Resources to promote health in positive terms must be identified and more fully mobilized. Art in its many patterns is one easily available resource that is generally unrecognized for its health-enhancing possibilities.[5] In order to learn more concretely what these benefits might be, I will examine drama, a major art form, and analyze its capacities for promoting health and improving health care.

First I think it would be helpful to look briefly at some basic qualities of art in general, as seen by philosophers, critics, and artists. One influential writer on aesthetics, R. G. Collingwood, argues that true art consists primarily of emotional expression and the stimulation of the imagination and that this contrasts with uses of art as craft, magic, amusement, and representation.[6] Emotions are liberated, focused, and communicated in art in ways that synthesize affective and cognitive functions; art enhances human imaginative capacities to make new symbols, forms, and interpretations of life.[7] Collingwood also states that the artist optimally constructs new images in active collaboration with his audience, so that artistic enterprises are in reality *community* experiences of creating new perceptions, values, and beliefs.[8] Life experiences for all participants are examined, focused, and intensified.[9]

Other dimensions of art promote health: art affirms the existence of the individual, as Nietzsche observed;[10] art gives the artist a sense of power to shape her world as she would like to experience it. Susanne Langer states that "that characteristic excitement [the aesthetic emotion], so closely wedded to original conception and inner vision, is not the source, but the effect, of artistic labor, the personal emotive experience of revelation, insight, mental power, which an adventure in 'implicit understanding' inspires."[11] This reformation or radical recreation can occur on various scales ranging from personal to universal. Furthermore, Nietzsche asserts that contrary to common opinion, "there is no such thing as pessimistic art; . . . art affirms."[12] Such a process that encourages emotional expression and creative imagination has positive, affirmative effects on health.

In contrast to the ideals expressed by scientists, art consciously promotes the process of incorporating feelings, values, and beliefs into the artistic product, as well as into the creative process. Subjective involvement is required to use objective techniques and materials. The literary artist must be personally engaged as he attempts to communicate a "message" that cannot be adequately expressed in other terms, beyond the limitation of words.[13] The artist must rely on intuitive, tacit knowledge. He knows "more than he can say."[14] In this sense art is mysterious, magical, and best experienced without effort to analyze and rationalize its components.

Some significant changes are taking place in medicine that tend to counteract the overwhelming emphasis on the scientific method as the only valid way to search for reality. The fallacy of looking for a single cause of disease has become obvious, as multiple psychological and cultural influences on illness have demonstrated. Few doubt the significance of psychosomatic mechanisms, usually found in hypertension, asthma, peptic ulcer, and many other diseases. Clinical practitioners are increasingly recognizing that they have only partial control of the conditions that alleviate disease. No longer can they suppose that most of the important events in healing are taking place in the hospital or clinic; the health professional must somehow travel with the patient back home to the family, neighborhood, and community where people live most of their lives. Primary responsibility for management of illness and wellness in most cases rests not with the health professional, but with the patient and family members, for they are the ones who make decisions within their own value and belief systems that fit their economic realities and cultural dynamics. At best the health professional is a valued but limited source of technical information. In times of acute crisis the practitioner may necessarily be the powerful authority figure who directs specific actions or technical procedures, but soon the primary authority returns to the individual, trusted relatives, and friends. A healthy self-esteem and strong self-confidence become major assets in recovery and the return to a satisfactory way of life. Psychiatry and behavioral sciences have led the way in recognizing the profound influence of self-image and identity in achieving progress in many physical and psychological problems.[15] The many dimensions of "personhood" in cultural and metaphysical terms thus become a valid concern for the student of health and health care.

But it is not only the personhood of the patient that is involved; the person of the practitioner is significant, too. The insights, experience, and integration of feelings, values, and beliefs are of crucial influence in the lives of health professionals as well. Furthermore, they must learn to function in a partnership with those who come for help in solving problems imaginatively and in creative ways.

Drama is an unusually fertile art form in which to explore relationships to health and health care for the professional and for the lay person. Drama is rich in subject matter, modes of presentation, and performance skills that can promote health, whether or not these are applied personally or in a formal health-care setting. Good theater usually is constructed around a problem which includes tension and conflict that are resolved in partially unpredictable ways. These situations often embody personal, community, cultural, and metaphysical issues shared by many people, with direct significance for health and illness, and of general societal concern.

Modern American dramatists have illuminated many contemporary problems that are related to disease. Eugene O'Neill, for example, in *Long Day's Journey into Night* writes about the interplay between chemical dependency and family dynamics, about his brother's and his own alcoholism, and about his mother's morphine addiction. If one studies O'Neill's artistic work in light of his personal life, medical history, and psychological development, he discovers powerful and subtle insights for people with these kinds of problems.[16] Almost inevitably the drama student or theatergoer will absorb affective and intellectual learning on a deep level and will find themes about life stages, death, and other diseases often included in many other well-known plays.[17]

Various aspects of family life have provided the subject matter for plays throughout theater history. The destructive effect of sibling rivalry has seldom been shown so clearly as in the relationship between Walter and Victor in Arthur Miller's *The Price*. The importance of the ongoing influence of their domineering, although deceased, father can be directly useful for professional and lay people who face comparable processes. Edward Albee brings an explicit awareness of the desperation, pain, and defeat in families similar to the one portrayed in *A Delicate Balance*. The reader or observer of Robert Anderson's *I Never Sang for my Father* learns dimensions of the father-son relationship that are difficult, if not impossible, to obtain from behavioral science analyses.

Many health processes look different when seen through cross-cultural lenses. This is especially true for the health professional who works with patients from ethnic, economic, or social backgrounds dissimilar to his own. In communities, definitions of wellness and illness may differ from neighborhood to neighborhood. Drama can provide a brief, intense immersion in another culture or social class.[18] In Miller's *A View from the Bridge* one learns something of the struggle for survival from members of an Italian immigrant community. Tennessee Williams allows viewers from middle and upper economic classes to experience some of the alienation and rejection, as well as satisfactions, experienced by working class people in *A Streetcar Named Desire*. The feelings and thoughts of a black youth who never knew his father are shared in Richard Wesley's *The Past is Past*.

Health and disease conditions are intimately connected with values and beliefs that are seldom examined at a deep level. These include political, religious, and philosophical assumptions that influence personal and professional lives in ways sometimes subtle but profound. Plays such as Lillian Hellman's *Watch on the Rhine* challenge viewers to examine their own political stance in respect to institutions and events close at hand, as well as those occurring internationally. Miller's *Death of a Salesman* can cause the reflective observer to ask what attitudes and actions are of his own choosing in contrast to accepting prevailing norms.

From the above sampling of subject material from contemporary drama, one can draw important lessons about prevalent disease conditions, family dynamics, cross-cultural phenomena, and values that influence health. There are other aspects of drama that are of significance to the promotion of health in general and to the learning of particular skills. One striking example is the use of improvisational drama for children in curricular and extracurricular settings, with a major objective being the enhancement of the young persons' emotional health, imaginative powers, and communication skills. Isabel Burger, who led this movement nationally, followed a sequence of learning that moved through pantomime, mood change, and dialogue to story situations.[19] At times these activities evolved into formal play productions such as Dickens's *A Christmas Carol*, but always the major emphasis was on problem-solving and on communicating feelings and thoughts effectively.[20]

Dramatic skills and ideas have been used by some experts studying family dynamics and practicing family therapy. Virginia Satir, a family therapist and well-known author, has concluded that certain roles typically played in family life lead to unhealthy relationships and sickness.[21] The "blamer" finds fault and induces guilt feelings. The "computer" or analyst attempts to take a purely cognitive or rational approach to all problems without allowing personal feelings to be expressed or accepted as important parts of the transaction. The "placator" constantly attempts to smooth over any disagreement or apparent conflict arising among family members. Often one family member tries to humor, act silly, or behave with irrelevance as a "distractor" in the home setting; tension is temporarily reduced by such tactics, but the underlying problem usually continues unimproved. Satir asks participants (or "patients," if in a medical setting) to play one of these roles in an imaginary family situation in which members seek to solve typical problems, such as planning for a holiday or disciplining a child. After undergoing the pain and frustration of these negative ways of communicating, she helps participants to learn new skills for acting in clear, direct, integral ways that enhance healthy family life.

Perhaps psychodrama is the most powerful form of theater consciously used for therapeutic and health promotional purposes. Participants simultaneously gain insight into themselves and invaluable skills for personal, public, and professional settings. In the 1920s J. L. Moreno was the innovator of this modality in which troublesome events or relationships in the life of the "protagonist" ("leading actor" or "patient") are reenacted.[22] The "director" (usually a health practitioner) assists the protagonist to describe the setting, situation, and plot, as he "warms up" to the acting process. Then with the help of supporting actors ("auxiliary egos"), who play family members or other significant persons, the "protagonist" is encouraged to act out the scene with spontaneity, intense emotional expression, and catharsis. Role reversal, soliloquy, doubling, and many other techniques are used. The group members support the "protagonist" throughout the process and in the closing period by speaking of their own responses to the story just enacted. Frequently parts of the drama are then reconstructed in ways that the protagonist would have preferred to have had the action develop. This basic design can be used in many ways in clinical, educational, and community settings. A group of caring, supportive people and a "director" with previous experience are essential and make possible experiences that are consistently helpful and therapeutic.

Sociodrama has many of the same elements as psychodrama, except that groups or communities act out situations where problems, conflicts, or tensions occur.[23] For a group or larger set of people, such as a school or community organization, sociodrama may be used without the connotation of "sickness" that is often associated with psychodrama. Closely akin to sociodrama is the performance of guerrilla theater, which uses theatrical devices to focus public attention on events or issues of political importance. Women's theater is employed for both political and aesthetic purposes. Group theater is another form in which interdependent improvisational acting is emphasized.[24]

Students are often introduced to their future careers by a variety of role-playing techniques. New or modified procedures in an ongoing employment setting are initiated and reinforced by this technique. Role models or supervisors demonstrate the desired behavior, which is often precisely described in procedure manuals or professional textbooks.[25] Great emphasis is placed on adherence to minute details of the "script." There is also a movement in professional education circles toward emphasizing problem-solving by the process of stating basic principles and then asking students to act out a unique, immediate response to the situation. This form of learning has proved valuable in training community health workers in developing countries where communication by nonverbal means is essential both for the health workers and the community workers.[26] Conflict, tension, and unpredictability are often intentionally planned in order to contribute to this kind of learning experience.

These experiences with dramatic techniques illustrate that drama and all the arts have potential value for health and health care far beyond what is currently being realized. For the communities of health professionals, artists, and for the public at large, however, a potentially disturbing question arises: How can experiences relating health and art be made more relevant, available, and integrated into the functions of each category—health practitioner, lay person, and artist? For medical service personnel the question can be broken down into areas with significant overlap: What are the benefits of education in the arts for personal growth? What are the helpful insights and experiences gained from art that are of aesthetic, cultural, social, and political concern and that broadly influence the directions of medical care and health? What particular skills, attitudes, and knowledge can be gained that will be useful in daily practice? Other questions are also certain to be asked: Are we suggesting that a major artistic element be introduced into a learning process currently dominated by science and technology? If so, at what stage—preprofessional, professional, or continuing education? What type of instruction would be necessary, and in what settings would these processes take place? Others might ask if such goals could not best be achieved by increasing the number and capacity of those specialists who currently use the arts as part of their therapy: music, dance, and art therapists; some psychiatrists; medical social workers; and health educators.

Let me address the last question first. It is obvious that there has been an increase in the kinds and number of therapists using music, dance, and the visual arts in health care. These new health practitioners are pioneering in the development of theoretical and practical knowledge that will probably have broader application in time to come.[27] But they seem to have constraints that currently limit their usefulness: they focus almost all their attention on acutely or seriously ill persons with major psychological or nervous system damage. This is understandable, since present use of the arts is largely limited to psychiatric settings. But "one does not have to be sick to get better," as the popular saying puts it, and the majority of people without serious illness could benefit as well. Although some psychiatrists do use psychodrama and other applications of the arts, psychiatric practice is confined primarily to individuals with clinical mental illness.

If indeed there are major health benefits to be derived from art, then art experiences must be available to more people than a small number of specialists can provide. Lay people and many kinds of health practitioners, particularly generalists, need to be involved in the interest of a wider influence and more effective health promotion. The preprofessional education of physicians, nurses, community health practitioners, and allied health personnel should be modified to include the contributions of the humanities and arts for health care specialists. To make such teaching effective, the instructors must give attention to both theoretical and practical relationships of the arts to health. Formal and informal study will help the teacher make appropriate application. Students and faculty will raise the continuing problem of competition for curricular time with the sciences. This reflects fundamental priority conflict and will take long and patient collaboration to resolve.

The professionalization process is a natural and important place to use the insights from art in health areas, because it is here that values, attitudes, and behavior are most deeply altered and imbedded. The ideal faculty for such teaching roles should have training and experience in both the arts and health care, although which should predominate is relatively unimportant, as long as the instructor can speak with authenticity from relevant experience. Since two to three hours of class time is enough for this kind of learning, this lessens the pressure on other areas for curriculum time. In the Health Associate Program at the Johns Hopkins University, primary care practitioners were educated for two years at the upper division baccalaureate level.[28] Students were allowed to choose from a variety of arts courses within the required curriculum. The student response was very positive, after some years of experimentation to find the most effective teaching forms.[29] I have developed courses in music, dance, and drama relating to health and health care that consistently evoke positive student response. One course entitled "Drama and Family Health" was offered for several years. Initially, plays including Miller's *The Price*, O'Neill's *Moon for the Misbegotten*, and Albee's *A Delicate Balance* were studied, discussed, and read in class in a kind of "readers theater." After studying and practicing Satir's family therapy techniques and Moreno's psychodrama ideas, students were invited to create a drama of their own clinical or personal experiences, using insights from all the above sources. Students almost always chose to develop scenes from their own family experiences, with classmates playing pertinent supporting roles. Each student also wrote a reflective paper that sought to synthesize his or her learning.

Postbasic continuing education connecting the arts and health provides many possible avenues to explore. Graduates learn as they work and are able to recognize more ways for the application of the arts than was possible during the initial professionalization process. The most effective situation for exploring these intersections is in conjunction with an ongoing health service center where teaching can be concrete. In a pioneering community center in southeast Baltimore, undergraduate, graduate, and continuing education students have been able to create dramatic events with lay people who collaborate in planning and performance. These plays have included disease and health-related topics such as alcoholism, aging, blindness, parent-child relationships, and neighborhood conflict. The health practitioners often provide technical information about disease, but neighborhood people supply the important knowledge about the social framework in which the events to be dramatized occur.

There is little doubt among the community center leaders that involvement in the arts brings new energy, imaginative insights, and opportunities for expression of feelings to the group that would not otherwise happen. Music, dance, and the visual arts are frequently incorporated into programs, with both amateur and professional artists involved. Specially planned coffeehouse evening events have combined poetry readings and music to address local and international issues such as racial and ethnic conflict, malnutrition, and resources for hope and optimism. An oil painting class led by a professional artist is producing some fine work by persons with almost no previous training. One woman who has suffered many difficult life crises, including the tragic loss of close family members, has taught herself to draw in crayon and watercolor, which has helped combat mental depression. She is so competent that several informal shows have been held, and a number of her pieces have been sold. The community center's interests in housing, social services, political activities, and social justice have been combined with health concerns. The arts are used in frequent festivals and celebrations that focus and highlight certain aspects of community life and promote heightened group consciousness, cohesion, and action.

The boundaries between laity, professionals, and amateurs are blurred or obliterated when health and art are approached in this way. The primary distinction of who is salaried becomes the main criterion for the term *professional.* Other rewards await the lay person who pursues art or health, or both. The original root meaning of *amateur*—one who engages in an activity for the love of it—is highly relevant; the "love" is closely bound up with the process of creating art, which makes the person feel good.

Professionals in both art and health are still needed by the community to perform, teach, and share skills, commitment, and knowledge. Obviously the skilled surgeon is essential to patients who need to have a surgical procedure. By the same token the professional violinist, painter, and choreographer are necessary to preserve classical works and to create the masterpieces that inspire the amateur artist and the participating community. Professionals in other disciplines also should give increased attention to the relationship of art and health, informing one another and making the benefits more understandable and obtainable. The philosopher can clarify aesthetic issues. The psychologist and physiologist can assist in elaborating on the mechanisms by which perceptions of form and symbol are transmitted into bodily functions. The health worker, however, probably holds the key role in consciously analyzing the dynamics of health and disease, which can be helped by appropriate artistic activities and in putting these insights into life-enhancing use. Educators in the health professions and the arts should be encouraged to experiment carefully and to innovate gradually; interested scholars, practitioners, and artists can contribute by developing and clarifying alternatives. All seek a common goal.

The best benefits will occur when effective partnerships develop between lay citizens and professionals in health and art. Then the patient not only becomes the "protagonist," but the lay person also gradually learns to be the "director" and eventually his own "playwright" for improved living. Prospects of well-being for all are enhanced, and new resources of imagination and emotional expression are harnessed for health.[30]

NOTES

1. The term *medicine* is used in this essay to include all the professional groups and their activities that deal with disease and health. Art in this discussion includes drama, music, dance, and the visual and plastic arts, or the "occurring arts," as Langer calls them. The relationship to the humanities is obviously close in many ways, but not the same.

2. The World Health Organization definition of health as "a state of complete physical, mental, and social well-being and not merely the absence of disease or infirmity" has withstood the criticism, and scorn at times, of those who consider it a meaningless ideal at best and usually a counterproductive illusion. Some efforts have been made by Eastern governments such as India to add the adjective denoting a spiritual dimension so that it would read "physical, mental, social, and spiritual well-being." This is particularly relevant when discussing artistic processes, since "spirit," "soul," and "ethos" are used frequently by critics and practitioners of the arts.

3. Susanne Langer has discussed many of the problems that limit the capacities of

the social and physical scientists in grappling with aesthetic issues in *Mind: An Essay on Human Feeling* (Baltimore, Md.: Johns Hopkins University Press, 1967), pp. 33–53.

4. "Doing Better and Feeling Worse: Health in the United States." *Daedalus,* Winter 1977. This entire issue is devoted to problems surrounding medical care: finances, ethics, distribution, education, research, and many other topics. In actuality when the term *health* is used it generally means *disease.*

5. The arts have been prominent in many traditional and classical cultures in many parts of the world. Sigerist wrote extensively about the relationships of medicine and music, visual arts, and literature in the mid-twentieth century in *Civilization and Disease* (Chicago: University of Chicago Press, 1943). Others have followed more recently such as George Rosen in *Madness in Society: Chapters in the Historical Sociology of Mental Illness* (New York: Harper and Row, 1968).

6. R. G. Collingwood, *the Principles of Art* (New York: Oxford University Press, 1938).

7. Langer, *Mind,* p. 27, n. 1. Langer quotes A. D. Ritchie's *The Natural History of the Mind* to say that "the essential art of thought is symbolization." Later she says "art may arise from almost any activity, and once it does so it is launched on a long road of explanation, invention, freedom to the limits of extravagance, interference to the point of frustration, finally discipline, controlling constant change and growth" (p. 143).

8. Collingwood, *Principles of Art,* pp. 300, n. 7. Langer also discusses commonalities of the artist and "beholder" (*Mind,* p. 259, n. 1).

9. See D'Arcy Hayman, *The Arts and Man* (Paris: UNESCO, 1969), pp. 11–25.

10. Friedrich Nietzsche, "The Will to Power," in *The European Philosophers: From Descartes to Nietzsche,* ed. Monroe C. Beardsley (New York: Random House, 1961), p. 869.

11. Langer, *Mind,* p. 259, n. 1.

12. Nietzsche, "The Will to Power," p. 869, n. 11.

13. See Louis O. Mink, *Mind, History, and Dialectic: The Philosophy of R. G. Collingwood* (Bloomington: Indiana University Press, 1969), p. 196. The classical view of art, and the dominant one through the Renaissance, was that art is a way of communicating knowledge that cannot be acquired or uttered in any other way.

14. See M. Polanyi, *Personal Knowledge: Towards a Post-Critical Philosophy* (Chicago: University of Chicago Press, 1958). Polanyi demonstrates how by "tacit" knowledge we know more than we can articulate in words.

15. Carl R. Rogers is one of the best known, but certainly not the only leading psychologist who has devoted much scholarship to the question of "personhood." See *On Becoming a Person* (Boston: Houghton Mifflin Co., 1961). Paul Tournier, a psychiatrist working in Switzerland, published widely on the subject in Europe. See *The Meaning of Persons* (New York: Harper and Row, 1957).

16. See Mink, *Mind, History, and Dialectic,* p. 207, n. 14. Mink holds that Collingwood does *not* believe that an artistic work can be better understood by reference to the biography of the artist. On the contrary, a careful study of O'Neill's life certainly seems to illuminate many otherwise obscure parts of his plays.

17. See Joanne Trautmann and Carol Pollard, *Literature and Medicine: Topics, Titles, and Notes* (Philadelphia: Society for Health and Human Values, 1975).

18. See C. J. Ducasse, "Art and the Language of the Emotions," in *Artistic Expression,* ed. John Hospers (New York: Appleton Century Crofts, 1971), p. 95. Tolstoy wrote in 1898, "Art is a human activity consisting in this, that one man consciously, by means of certain external signs, hands on to others feelings he has lived through, and that other people are infected by these feelings, and also experience them." Tolstoy, *What is Art?* (London: Oxford, 1899).

19. Isabel Burger, *Creative Playacting: Learning Through Drama* (New York: Ronald Press, 1966).

20. See Joanna Halpert Kraus, "Children's Theatre, Baltimore Style," *Players* 47 (1971): 204–9.

21. Virginia Satir, *Conjoint Family Therapy: A Guide to Theory and Technique* (Palo Alto, Calif.: Science and Behavior Books, 1964); V. Satir, *Peoplemaking* (Palo Alto, Calif.: Science and Behavior Books, 1972).

22. J. L. Moreno and Z. T. Moreno, *Psychodrama* (Beacon, N.Y.: Beacon House, 1975), vol. 3: *Action Therapy and Principles of Practice;* Ira A. Greenberg, ed., *Psychodrama: Theory and Therapy* (New York: Behavioral Publications, 1974).

23. See Moreno and Moreno, *Psychodrama,* p. 270.

24. See. B. Clark, *Group Theatre* (New York: Theatre Arts Books, 1971); S. Elkind, *Improvisational Handbook* (Glenview, Ill.: Scott, Foresman & Co., 1975): J. Hodgson and E. Richards, *Improvisation* (London: Eyre Methuen Ltd., 1974).

25. See D. Schecter and T. M. O'Farrell, eds., *Training and Continuing Education: A Handbook for Health Care Institutions* (Chicago: Hospital Research and Educational Trust, 1970).

26. See Y. F. Tarfa, "Basic Health Services for Rural Areas in Nigeria," in R. W. McNeur, ed., *The Changing Roles and Education of Health Care Personnel Worldwide in View of the Increase of Basic Health Services* (Philadelphia: Society for Health and Human Values, 1978), pp. 69–80.

27. See E. T. Gaston, *Music in Therapy* (New York: Macmillan Co., 1968); E. Rosen, *Dance in Psychotherapy* (New York: Dance Horizons Republication, 1974); S. Chaiklin, "Dance Therapy," in S. Arieto, ed., *American Handbook of Psychiatry* (New York: Basic Books, 1975.); L. Gantt and M. S. Schmal, *Art Therapy: A Bibliography* (Rockville, Md.: National Institute of Mental Health, 1974).

28. See A. S. Golden, D. G. Carlson, and H. L. Hagen, eds., *The Art of Teaching Primary Health Care* (New York: Springer, 1981).

29. See my "The Humanities and Arts in Primary Health Care Education," in Golden, et al., *The Art of Teaching Primary Health Care.* This chapter presents an overview of the conceptual framework and actual operation of this humanities and arts program.

30. See G. Berg, D. Carlson, E. Fee, S. Gadow and L. Hunt, "Humanistic Studies in the Health Associate Program: Revisions and New Directions," in R. K. McElhinney, ed., *Human Values Teaching Programs for Health Professionals: Self-Descriptive Reports from Twenty-Nine Schools* (Philadelphia: Society for Health and Human Values, 1976).

"How Annandale Went Out"— A Doctor's Decision

PETER GRAHAM

Virginia Polytechnic Institute and State University

> "They called it Annandale—and I was there
> To flourish, to find words, and to attend:
> Liar, physician, hypocrite, and friend,
> I watched him; and the sight was not so fair
> As one or two that I have seen elsewhere:
> An apparatus not for me to mend—
> A wreck, with hell between him and the end,
> Remained of Annandale; and I was there.
>
> "I knew the ruin as I knew the man;
> So put the two together, if you can,
> Remembering the worst you know of me.
> Now view yourself as I was, on the spot—
> With a slight kind of engine. Do you see?
> Like this . . . You wouldn't hang me? I thought not."

Edwin Arlington Robinson's "How Annandale Went Out" is a dramatic monologue that persistently fascinates and perplexes its readers. The poem proves as efficient as it is enigmatic. Within the scope of a sonnet's octave and sestet its speaker, a physician at the bedside of a dying friend, resolves a complex moral problem: he decides to commit euthanasia. The general progression of events seems clear enough—at poem's end Annadale has indeed "gone out" with the speaker's active assistance—but the particulars of method and motive remain disconcertingly vague. We must ask the right questions to decipher the truths Robinson half states and half conceals.

Many readers out to solve Robinson's riddle focus on Annandale, the passive member of the doctor-patient relation, in hopes of learning what the dying man suffers from and what purchases his release. "Annandale Again," a sequel that appeared twenty-two years after "How Annandale Went Out," suggests that the agony resulted from an automobile or carriage accident: "There was a sick crash in the street, / And after that there was no doubt / Of what there was. . . ."[1] But in the earlier poem Robinson specifies neither the patient's condition nor the means employed to change it, so those who seek a diagnosis or autopsy for Annandale remain conjecturers. Other readers who find this first approach less than fruitful discuss "How Annandale Went Out" in light of resemblances between the poem's situation and the poet's experience.[2] Although it is interesting to learn that Robinson's older brother, Dean, a physician addicted to opiates, apparently died of a self-administered overdose of morphine, such knowledge cannot indicate just where the poet's personal response to a real tragedy ends and imaginative projection begins.

Ultimately, pondering the mysterious author or his unknowable title character distracts us from what certainty can be discovered in the poem. Only by remaining where Robinson places us, within the consciousness of his speaker, can we trace the pattern in the web of words. Scrutinizing the physician brings ample rewards. We come to understand one man's mind, see how his attitudes reflect the medical thought of his day, and discover from his judgment an empirical answer to one of medicine's most difficult questions—the dilemma of euthanasia.

Robinson's background enabled him to depict a contemporary physician convincingly. Since his admired brother was a doctor and his family suffered more than their fair share of serious illness, alcoholism, and drug addiction, Robinson possessed a certain familiarity with medical matters. He kept his brother's copy of Sir Richard Quain's *Dictionary of Medicine* among his personal books: this retention may have been a matter of sentiment but may suggest that the poet's interest in medicine was more than casual.[3] Certainly reading Sir Thomas Browne, whose *Urn-burial* he pronounced "magnificent,"[4] offered Robinson a precedent for joining art and diagnosis. Like Browne, the doctor-speaker Robinson depicts in "How Annandale Went Out" possesses verbal talents comparable to his medical expertise.

David Nivson has noted that "How Annandale Went Out"

differs from most of Robinson's other dramatic monologues in being entirely enclosed by quotation marks. This punctuation might indicate that one speaker is reporting another's words.[5] Or, as I would like to argue, it might emphasize that the reader must pay close attention to the exact words before him. Certainly a careful appraisal of diction proves necessary in the octave's tableau of physician and patient, where we discern the situation, prognosis, and speaker's character less from the facts presented than from the phrases chosen to convey them. Although obvious medical allusions appear nowhere in the poem, the speaker's insights and expressions obliquely reveal him as a thoughtful and articulate turn-of-the-century man of science. For instance, the phrase he uses to signify his bedside responsibilities—"To flourish, to find words, and to attend"—seems evasive but functions precisely. The verbs chosen sidestep the explicit, as does substitution of "went out" for the more usual "died" in the title, but accurately convey the complex, almost antagonistic demands placed on one who is "liar, physician, hypocrite, and friend" to the dying Annandale. As a medical man the "flourishing" speaker makes professional passes over his patient; as "flourishing" friend he survives and thereby perpetuates in his memory a man already departed from a failing body. The physician "finds words" that name Annandale's problem; the liar, hypocrite, and friend find others that comfort and conceal. Likewise, friend and physician "attend" in different ways: the first awaits what is inevitable; the second will do what can be done. At this point, however, even medical attendance involves observation rather than action. The doctor "watches," and we watch him watching. He assesses the gravity of his patient's condition. As he articulates his findings, we gauge his sensibility.

The doctor's references to Annandale as "it," "apparatus," "wreck," and "ruin" dehumanize as efficiently as the current clinical jargon, "terminal case," would do. In describing his patient as a machine the doctor speaks in accord with the intellectual spirit of his age. With the rise of scientific medicine and the germ theory in the 1870s, practitioners became able to identify disease-causing organisms. Focusing on what could be seen with certainty, they tended to reduce the patient to his complaint. But Robinson's doctor has a more conscious reason for speaking of Annandale as he does. Annandale *is* inanimate. The case is hopeless; the spirit has fled. The physician understands that his former comrade has become "an apparatus not for me to mend." We may suspect from these words, which strongly echo the unfavorable verdict ("An ailment not to be treated") appended to the diagnoses of incurable complaints by the ancient Egyptian physicians, the speaker's awareness of the medical practices recorded in the papyri, traditions made more generally accessible by the 1890 translation of the Papyrus Ebers into German.[6] Locating Annandale's hell "between him and the end," the doctor reverses the Christian order of events and subjectively focuses on the suffering that his profession treats, the mortal pain that ends with earthly life. From his clinical perspective, Annandale must have nothing to lose and everything to gain by his death. Thus, apparently offhand words and phrases show what scientific training, scholarly interests, and personal convictions the doctor-speaker brings to the situation confronting him. We have learned how he thinks and shall see how he acts.

The octave and sestet of "How Annandale Went Out" contrast in several ways. In the two divisions of his dramatic monologue the speaker offers complementary temporal perspectives on the crucial action that takes place offstage. The octave provides, as we have noted, a *mise en scène;* the sestet justifies the *fait accompli.* Hence the speaker makes different demands on his audience in the two sections and modulates his tone accordingly. In the octave, which describes the tentative phase before the doctor commits himself to a course of action, he asks only that we examine the facts of the case objectively. His exposition may predispose us in his favor, but we watch him from the outside. Tentativeness and objectivity vanish in the sestet. His die cast, the speaker desires our sanction. He seeks it subjectively, by drawing us into his mind. The rhetoric of direct address makes us partners in his mental process of self-justification, and by the end of the poem he counts on our complicity.

But despite their differing purposes, techniques, and tones, the two parts of the poem have the same context. The sestet, like the octave, carefully locates doctor and patient in history and shows Robinson's awareness of the state of medicine at the turn of the century. Imaginatively reenacting the "missing center" of his story, the doctor admits that he has released Annandale from death-in-life through the agency of what he coyly calls "a slight kind of engine," probably a hypodermic syringe, a device that first gained wide use when opiates were introduced in the nineteenth century. By merely increasing the dosage of the narcotic he would very likely be injecting to dull his patient's pain, the doctor could humanely and inconspicuously ease Annandale over the threshold.

However the deed is done, in deciding to commit active euthanasia—helping, rather than merely permitting his patient to die—the physician embraces the most radical solution to a problem that doctors and laymen alike had begun to consider seriously in the 1870s.[7] Advances in medical science had enabled physicians to sustain life with ever-increasing success. This new power brought with it fresh uncertainties that continue to puzzle modern medicine. What should the doctor do when his responsibility to sustain life conflicts with his duty to ease suffering? How far should medicine go in easing or even hastening an inevitable and agonizing death? Many people, among them the *Boston Medical and Surgical Journal* writer who argued in 1906 for active euthanasia in the cases of patients reduced to "nothing but the external form with its associations of memory to show that it has been the abiding place of a soul now evicted,"[8] saw a comfortable death as something that humane, conscientious physicians could and should provide.

In "How Annandale Went Out" active euthanasia ends the physician's suffering along with his patient's. The doctor presented in the octave is a confused man in search of an appropriate role. As the poem begins, authority rests with an unnamed aggregate of outsiders; the speaker's medical relation to his patient is mere juxtaposition: "They called it Annandale—and I was there." The doctor knows that in this situation he cannot heal as the voice of society enjoins. What then can he do but equivocate? The beginning of the sestet, in contrast, rings with authority: "I knew the ruin as I knew the man." As a physician, the speaker understands what Annandale's mishap has left him; as a friend he recalls what Annandale once was. A cryptic imperative for action follows in the next line: "So put the two together, if you can." "Put the two together"—what two? Obviously the present and the former Annandales are irreconcilable. The speaker, though, can unite two disjointed aspects of his own being, his medical training and his personal empathy, in the convention-defying act of euthanasia. So doing, he discards the roles of liar and hypocrite that encumbered him in the octave. Before stating his action more explicitly, the speaker asks us to second-guess him, "Remembering the worst you know of me." This warning is his artful disavowal of rhetorical art. The best and worst we know of the speaker is what he chooses to tell us. We have seen him as a caring friend, a watchful diagnostician, an unorthodox theologian, and a scholar able to take the long view of his profession. The worse we know, then, (if, as he implies, we belong to the conformist majority) is that the speaker can dispense with our conventions. But because we have participated sympathetically in the formation of his judgment, we grant in context the approval we might otherwise withhold. The speaker's final words, "You wouldn't hang me? I thought not," show his awareness of having won his point. He has brought his audience to a situational understanding, perhaps even acceptance, of active euthanasia.

In "How Annandale Went Out" Robinson gives a moral position situational qualifications, embodies it in an individuated mind, and frames position, situation, and mind within an historical context. Then he clouds the facts. To read them right we must exercise some of the diagnostic dexterity that enables the physician-speaker sensitively to assist his dying friend. Thus as we elucidate the poem we walk a path that parallels the speaker's medical and ethical explorations. "How Annandale Went Out" enables us to trace an etiology of euthanasia and to pronounce the physician who commits it healthy.

Timely though the contexts of "How Annandale Went Out" may be, its lesson is a timeless one. In pondering and then solving the problem before him, the poem's speaker avoids the extreme positions that are equally inappropriate for men and women of medicine. He neither reduces himself to a technician, a mere appendage of medical science, nor raises himself to a godlike decider of destiny, as does the Faustian protagonist of Shaw's *The Doctor's Dilemma. "Ni ange ni bîte,"* Robinson's doctor remembers his own humanity and that of his friend and patient: he lives and acts in that Pascalian middle world where all man's ethical choices must be made.

NOTES

1. Edwin Arlington Robinson, *Collected Poems* (New York: MacMillan, 1959), p. 1200.

2. See in particular David S. Nivson, "Does It Matter How Annandale Went Out?" in *An Appreciation of Edwin Arlington Robinson*, ed. Richard Cary (Waterville, Maine: Colby College Press, 1969), pp. 178–90.

3. James Humphrey, *The Library of Edwin Arlington Robinson* (Waterville, Maine: Colby College Press, 1950), p. 41. I am also grateful to J. Fraser Cocks III of the Colby College Library, for additional information concerning Robinson's copy of Quain's *Dictionary of Medicine*.

4. Edwin Arlington Robinson, *Untriangulated Stars: The Letters of Edwin Arlington Robinson to Harry DeForest Smith, 1890–1905*, ed. Denham Sutcliffe (Cambridge, Mass.: Harvard University Press, 1947), p. 124.

5. Nivson, "Does It Matter," p. 185.

6. Henry E. Sigerist, *A History of Medicine*, 2 vols. (New York: Oxford University Press, 1951), 1:306–10. Though no German scholar, Robinson had studied the language at Harvard in 1892–93 (Robinson, *Untriangulated Stars*, pp. 71, 76, 84, 86, 90, 117). Hence he should have been able to read the Papyrus Ebers translation.

7. Stanley J. Reiser, "The Dilemma of Euthanasia in Modern Medical History: The English and American Experience," in *Ethics and Medicine: Historical Perspectives and Contemporary Concerns*, ed. Stanley J. Reiser, Arthur J. Dyck, and William J. Curran (Cambridge, Mass.: MIT Press, 1977), p. 488.

8. "Euthanasia—Degenerated Sympathy," *Boston Medical and Surgical Journal* 154(1906): 330–31, quoted in Reiser et al., *Ethics and Medicine*, p. 490.

Pathos and Pathology: Physicians in *The Last Angry Man*, *M*A*S*H*, and *The Magician*

EDMUND L. ERDE

New Jersey School of Osteopathic Medicine

> I say it is a just cause of complaint that when we, the priests, have left off the worship of Baal, and have deserted the groves and high places, and have sworn allegiance to the true god of science, that you, the people, should wander off after all manner of idols, and delight more and more in patent medicines, and be more than ever at the hands of advertising quacks. But for a time it must be so. This is yet the childhood of the world, and a supine credulity is still the most charming characteristic of man.
>
> Some of the brightest hopes of humanity are with the medical profession. To it, not to law or theology, belong the promises.
>
> William Osler, "Recent Advances in Medicine"

The appendix of this essay[1] describes the plots of three films—*The Last Angry Man,*[2] *M*A*S*H,*[3] and *The Magician*[4]—that portray doctors and other helpers of people. The reader who is unfamiliar with these films or who has a vague recollection of them may wish to read the appendix before sections 1 and 2. Section 1 analyzes the themes and symbols of these films in juxtaposition to one another. Section 2 discusses the moral, cultural, and historical concepts implicit in the films and relates the details in the film criticism to contemporary medicine.

This project is important for several reasons. Stories give direction to and exemplify the applications of moral slogans and maxims, which is essential for the slogans and maxims to be meaningful.[5] Further, people seem to prefer representations to reality; producing and consuming images is a major cultural activity. Moreover, images reflect and determine our demands and expectations. Indeed, even today humans waver between distinguishing images from real things and feeling the magical tie of images to their objects.[6]

1

The humanist-physician, Felix Marti-Ibanez, confronts us with a dichotomy. He writes, "The pendulum of the physician's professional thinking swings between two dangers: magic and [unscientific] dogmatism."[7] What is true of the physician may be true for the profession as well. Thus, the dichotomy stands as a challenge for us to choose between defining the essence of medicine in terms of pathos (the magic that Vogler offers in *The Magician*) or pathology (the science of Vergerus in *The Magician* and the *M*A*S*H* surgeons).

But the three films show the choice to be more complex than this, for in them we find *three* ways of conceiving physicians, the practice of medicine, and patients. *M*A*S*H* shows doctors as surgeons, as masters of physical technique; their patients are bodies. *The Last Angry Man* presents the doctor as rational, concerned with disease and dignity; the doctor presumes his patients to be rational minds and bodies. *The Magician* portrays all persons as patients and all patients as bodies having minds with spiritual and symbolic needs.

In spite of the choices being more than two, the halves of Marti-Ibanez's dichotomy have traditional, symbolic, and thematic associations (not all of which wind up as clear opposites) that dominate a great deal of thinking about humans and medicine.

The choices can be cast in symbolic terms based upon the mythic gods of Greece—Dionysus and Apollo. Dionysus symbolizes participating in the furious, wild forces of nature; Apollo symbolizes the cold, removed, analytical ability to intervene in nature.[8] The former has also been associated with the god Pan.[9] As doctors, persons of this cast would be pathos-oriented. They seem warm, intimate, careless, or imprecise persons who understand and appreciate nature; they work with it rather than intervene against it. They rely neither on logic nor scientific technique. Instead, they rely on their understanding of "the wisdom of the body" and participate fully in nature—in being sexual, dirty or grubby, wild, coarse, noisy, unscientific, and overpowering. They practice holistic medicine and they live actively and use the forces of nature with subtlety, as magicians, as intuitive (even perhaps blind) mediators between patients and the nature of which they partake. The Apollonians, by contrast, are the pathologists. They seem cold, aloof, astere, clinical, clean, and detached from nature but involved in science and technology. These people intervene. They themselves seem mechanical yet more godlike than human. Everything such healers do would be deliberate in contrast with the intuitive, causal actions of their opposites.

Another set of symbolic categories that might be brought to bear on the physician include the "Wounded Healer" and the "Trickster." Guggenbuhl-Craig describes it this way:

> There are some individuals who are so fascinated by the eternal struggle between sickness and health that they feel called upon to take part in that battle. They do not wish to avoid it or merely suffer it passively.[10]

Being a wounded healer is possible for either Appollonian or Dionysian physicians, but such persons can go astray, perhaps as Sam Abelman (the last angry man) does, in not recognizing that the battle and the need for battle can occur on all three levels: body, mind, and spirit. Or the struggle can go astray in thinking it has to be fought solely on scientific grounds.

Carl Jung might say that one way such persons could go astray would be to lose contact with the dual ingredients of their nature—by thinking of themselves as healers and repressing their awareness of their own wounds. At this point, the notion of the Trickster comes to the fore. Jung tells us that the Trickster represents the primitive (undifferentiated) human who is hardly beyond the animal level, and who, though an unruly rogue, can heal.[11] Indeed, the Trickster is coextensive with the shaman and medicine man and shares with them the fact that practicing their craft puts them in danger and involves much suffering (being *wounded*-healers). But it is appropriate to caution against over simplifying Jung's thought. Almost every figure that he discusses has phases of development and a good and a bad (shadow) side. In some phases, the Trickster is demonic and unpredictable, inadvertently leaving destruction in his wake through sly pranks.[12] In other phases, he gradually evolves into a saintly or saviorlike figure.[13] Thus, we might say that when the wounded-healer goes astray by forgetting his own woundedness, he can become a destructive Trickster.

The healers may set out to be followers of the destructive Trickster, or they may just wind up that way. Those who set out to be quacks might choose that form of embezzlement because unconsciously they are responsive to the wounded-healer within. People who just wind up as followers of the destructive Trickster may be destructive in their medical practice, or they may be destructive in other aspects of their lives. If they are destructive practicing medicine, then they fulfill just what the rational Apollonian opposes in an irrational Dionysian. That is, the rational Apollonians oppose well-intended quackery that they presume to rely upon no science. But then the Apollonians seem to identify no science (art?) with false science. They then go on to identify false science with nonmechanistic science. Thus they come to oppose the Dionysian. The follower of Apollo opposes embezzlers and Dionysians indifferently, as happens in *The Magician. M*A*S*H* represents a different conflict, a conflict between destructive Tricksters outside of medical practice. Within medicine the heroes in *M*A*S*H* are the cold priests of technology. They can cause panic in most other contests, and they are themselves victimized by those aspects of themselves (Pan, Trickster, Wounded-Healer) with which they are out of touch. Still, the film implies that trying to restrict the antics of nonprofessional activities fails; the trickster energy leaks into medical relationships.

For Jung, though, there is a positive potential to the shadow-figures, the negative complement of the common sense aspect of mind. Such shadow-figures can be confronted, understood, and befriended. Indeed they can be useful allies.[14] Trouble arises only from those who repress the shadow-figure, for this alienates humans from aspects of themselves and may force persons and society to construct scapegoats whereby the shadow is personified and incarnated.[15]

Let me combine the above points about wounds and Tricksters this way. The Trickster within each person is a wound for those who identify themselves as rationalists. If Jung is right, such people believe that logic alone can solve all (or all solvable) problems.[16] They are out of touch with the human dimension that connects us with more than information and information processing—the part of us that needs a Dionysian physician. Our human needs include myth and symbolic enactments, but the rationalist believes logic and motor control or technological technique can fulfill all requirements. It is tempting to say that the Dionysian and the Trickster are on one side of a divide and indeed are complements of one another. It is more helpful, however, to suggest that each symbol is an ingredient or dimension of the personality of each of us.

In the time in which *The Magician* is set, one nagging question was whether there could be a science of animal magnetism. There was a great feud between those who believed in a vitalist theory of life—the belief that some vital substance animated matter to make it alive—and those who believed the antithesis, that all life could be explained by anatomical functioning of matter that was perfectly mechanical. Indeed, the struggle between Vogler and Vergerus could be symbolic of Mesmer's life story or even of the broader struggle of the time.[17] But as *The Magician* shows that the scientist can be humbled by his broader needs, *The Last Angry Man* shows that the physician who is insensitive to these needs in his patients will not have many patients. *M*A*S*H* shows that the wounded healer and the Trickster will haunt even the powerful technocrat in ways that are very disquieting, even to the technocrats.

In these three portraits of healers, then, the Apollonian and Dionysian ingredients are distributed in strikingly different ways. Sam, the former athlete, is of Dionysus-Pan in his worship of nature, in his anger, and in his interpersonal patient relationships. The *M*A*S*H* men, the antiheroes, are Dionysian in their lack of esteem for the military social order, in their ability to cause panic in their enemies, in their dress, in their sexuality, and in their debauchery. But they are also Apollonian priests of technology and can sustain a separate social order where technical competence controls, even within the context of the Korean War.

Vogler sends mixed messages. He is elegantly dressed and clean except for travel dust. He seems to be an abstainer; he is silent—feigning to be mute; he seems to be unattached, even celibate—though his wife is present in disguise. He boasts that his craft is scientific and disavows such things as the force of personality—though he does seem to have special powers. Indeed, his special powers are of Pan, and they evoke panic from Vergerus. If the magician heals all, he does so through the emotions.

Of the three, only Vogler understands the psyche and ritual. The *M*A*S*H* men have become like Vergerus; none of them believes in ritual at all. Vergerus comes as close as he can to a ritual by performing an autopsy. The *M*A*S*H* men meet ritual with antics.[18] Sam would at best meet ritual with silent, impatient tolerance, but more typically he would meet it with anger. Vogler, as magician, is himself a symbol. In being wounded (mute), in being mysterious (claiming magical power), in being a Christ-figure (there is much relevant symbolism in the film), he becomes a catalyst or an occasion to which the established social order must respond with either belief and healing compliance or with anger and harassment. (Perhaps this is so because medicine itself would be too insecure to allow society to remain indifferent to one of its challengers.)

Each type of physician portrayed in the three films suffers. Sam's anger and youthful attempted suicide make his wounds obvious; most obvious of all is his dying at the end while giving a detailed description of his symptoms. The military physicians suffer as well. They, too, must act out their suffering. The one among them who actually is hurting, the dentist who thinks he has become impotent, receives mock ritual in the well-known Last Supper scene. In it, he is attempting suicide, but the physicians have contrived to give him a placebo instead of a lethal drug. They trick their "patient" back to life but display little awareness of their own suffering. The magician knows a great deal about suffering. When he is out of his costume and with his wife, when his beard and longer hair and greater stature come off after the autopsy, he is a small, sheepish man who suffers from his sheepishness.

Thus, the three kinds of healers shown are wounded healers. But each is in tune with the depth of wound in a very different way. The plumbers of the body, the military surgeons, seem almost totally unaware of their wounds. The realistic, common sensical man, Dr. Abelman, at the end is aware of his physical wounds, as he had been aware in his youth of other kinds of suffering. The magician, the man who is a Trickster in his healing practice, speaks to needs and aspects of wounded patients in an altogether richer way than the other two. He speaks to the sickness of a soul and the sickness of a time. He, like Abelman, is angry, but he keeps his anger quiet and hopes that it will teach through nonrational means. Still, when he is alone, his suffering is manifest.

2

One implicit theme in these works involves the meaning, use, and importance of artistic representations of medicine. For one example, consider the effectiveness of instruction in or exposure to the humanities and the arts for the moral improvement of people. Assessments about such effectiveness vary from discounting the prospects entirely[19] to lauding the undertaking as definitely therapeutic.[20] For another example, one can debate the validity of human or moral implications built into positions taken on the basis of a work of fiction, because, in being a work of fiction, it can be a setup for a moral thesis. Is the occasion created to examine human experience in unfamiliar or crafted structures of moral significance?

Portrayals of the physician in drama or novels or film can, at the least, be taken to state what authors think of medicine and doctors or what they believe those persons with various backgrounds and cultures—some of which may resemble ours (if there is "one" of ours) and some of which may not—think about medicine and doctors. For example, in a 1979 *New York Times* essay,[21] Mel Gussow explored what he terms "The Time of the Wounded Hero." He was writing about a set of then-current plays that involved main characters stricken in their prime and confined to a wheelchair, a bed, or an iron lung—like "a modern Prometheus." Gussow takes the copresence of these plays to be more than coincidence. He quotes Leslie Fiedler's *Freaks* to the effect that such marginal beings seem to be a metaphor of our age: that premature death or premature incapacity reigns in our thoughts. Although Gussow also cites Amitai Etzioni's idea that the trend of writing about wounded heroes is an expression of a depressed society, he does not mention how the boom in medicine might itself be a consequence of this larger sense of incapacity.

These literary portraits of patients are very different from earlier renditions of medical encounters in which the doctor would be a principal character. Even Rudolph Virchow, the great nineteenth-century medical theorist and humanist, cared about the standard presentation of the physician in literature. He commented—or rather bemoaned—that most novels about physicians made them out to be deplorable figures.[22] Several historical studies[23] imply that the deplorable characters mentioned by Virchow were, by and large, cast as comic figures, really as buffoons. But in the last hundred years doctors (rather than patients) have assumed the role of hero[24]—a concept more closely associated with tragedy than comedy. Recently some thoughtful writing has characterized medicine's practice in the language of tragedy.[25] Tragedy results when physicians have to choose between conflicting right actions or conflicting wrongs.

The Last Angry Man is clearly a tragedy; Sam's heroic, righteous anger is in response to disease and irrationality. He is confronting the right value issues and is distressed by the limitations of his role and aware of the limitations of, and conflicts within, our existence. Yet as a physician he aims to sustain that existence. Being dead serious about himself as a physician, as Sam Abelman was, bodes decline and failure for a noble character. As a tragic hero, then, this doctor is an important symbol.

*M*A*S*H* is also a modern literary presentation of physicians, but it seems more akin to comedy than to tragedy. However, it is even more modern than *The Last Angry Man* because it is about antiheroes; rather than merely ridiculing physicians, as did older works, *M*A*S*H* is iconoclastic while acknowledging the technical mastery of the surgeons.

Whether *The Magician* is a comedy or a tragedy is not easy to decide. Its subtitle bills itself as a comedy. While the film does contain some jokes played upon characters, one or two funny moments, and some dashes of young love, it is much more like an existential horror movie until the end when the favorite protagonists are saved (as per *deus ex machina*) by a summons from the king. Set (by coincidence?) in the year (1958) that Rudolph Virchow believes he put an end to any scientific basis for a general or systematic or whole-person organization theory of pathology,[26] *The Magician* symbolizes an ideal in a moving way. The implied ideal is to add more magic to the modern doctor.[27] The more profound symbolism of the film, though, is that it has a power to move and to heal. This film tries to move each of us to find the wounds and the magician within ourselves.[28] *The Last Angry Man* tries to display or even convince us about the ideal physician (while showing the incommensurability of the ideal with the real). *The Magician* tries to harness elements within us that could not be called rational but could be called human nature. It tries to use these sensitivities and powers toward a healing of the viewer. We may "get ourselves together," then, through watching it; and we may get along with our business in a better though still ragtag way.

This is the key to why *The Magician* is a comedy. The formal trappings of comedy are present but hidden: the film begins at sunset and ends in the morning, the good guys win, and so on. But more than this, *The Magician* works on the viewer in the manner of comedy and diffuses the forces and demands of too much commitment to rationality.

Cavell has distinguished the comedy of Buster Keaton from that of Charlie Chaplin according to how each pursues and wins a degree of happiness.[29] Keaton wins through "outward aptness" or conscientiousness, keeping his poise no matter what happens to his plans. Chaplin wins through "inward aptness" or playfulness and imagination. These types of comedy can be mapped onto a set of categories borrowed from Conrad Hyers's *Zen and the Comic Spirit*.[30] Consider the level of innocent play of the child (living in a Paradise), the bitter, sarcastic joke of the sharp-tongued wit (activity in a Paradise Lost), and the mild, gentle, wise humor of the sage (living in a Paradise Regained). Keaton is funny for us where *we* live—in Paradise Lost. Chaplin is funny for us at both of the other levels. He is both childlike and instructive about how we may gather our spirits.

The angry doctor in *The Last Angry Man* and the film itself are not comic; but if they do affect us in the comic mode, it is in Keaton's conscientious vein. The people in *M*A*S*H* are imaginative; thus they are Chaplinesque. But they are also cruel and achieve outer but no inner aptness. Further, *M*A*S*H* does not help us to our own aptness of either kind. Thus, if it is a comedy, *M*A*S*H* is a degenerate comedy. But the humorless (except for Granny) people in *The Magician* can help us gather our inner spirit even as the magician follows Keaton's lead and, for the most part, keeps his own outer aptness.

This comic perspective may help explain why, as in *M*A*S*H,* today's doctors and today's priests seem to ignore one another or are pitted against one another, with the doctor far and away having the upper hand. It may also suggest two other points: how the battle is best conceived as a costly farce because both the medical priest (the physician) and the religious priest unknowingly miss the third party in their games—the tricky Pan—and why *The Magician* is billed as a comedy.

In "The Social Control of Cognition: Some Factors in Joke Perception," the anthropologist Mary Douglas compares Henri Bergson's theory of jokes to that of Freud. Bergson finds in humor a demonstration that intuition is superior to logic and that life transcends mechanism. For him the joke is an attack by a preferred value upon a lesser value: something that ridicules the mechanical view of man. Freud, though, believes wit gives the unconscious and the censor a holiday. By bringing different, even conflicting ideas into juxtaposition with an economy and charm that reduces the threat in the conflict, a joke thereby reduces the efforts of the censor. Douglas favors Freud's view because she thinks that Bergson cannot account for puns and other forms of humor. Still, she finds a level of agreement between them:

> For both the essence of the joke is that something formal is attacked by something informal, something organised and controlled, by something vital, energetic, an upsurge of life for Bergson, of libido for Freud. The common denominator underlying both approaches is the joke seen as an attack on control.[31]

And she summarizes her account of jokes thus:

> The joke merely affords opportunity for realizing that an accepted pattern has no necessity. Its excitement lies in the suggestion that any particular ordering of experience may be arbitrary and subjective. It is frivolous in that it produces no real alternative, only an exhilarating sense of freedom from form in general.[32]

Douglas then distinguishes standard jokes, in which the verbal form totally communicates that a joke is being made, from a spontaneous joke, which organizes the total situation in its pattern. Both of these joke forms are assaults, and when medicine and medical knowledge are the targets (as in *The Magician*, but not in *M*A*S*H*), the joke can be seen to subvert the accepted patterns that doctors take so seriously. That is why *The Magician* goes to the core of what medicine is about, and it is why some physicians are so thoroughly set against magic. Like Sam, like the *M*A*S*H* crew, like Vergerus, they presume that they know the true and necessary order of things and that they know its method—science—very well.[33] Still, one cannot help wondering whether even the more limited Bergsonian concept of a joke is not totally at one with the enterprise of medicine, which is to affirm vitality.[34]

The broader cultural and moral implications of this discussion are many, but they bear most directly on the concept of professionalism. The definition of professionalism is controversial, but, as Friedson has shown,[35] medicine is a profession in that its members have an expertise that others cannot judge well. In this sense the medical profession is at odds with the lay public. Thus, the following presumed tensions are stressful, although perhaps they grant too much credence to professional judgment: (a) Strain results when some physicians try to be responsive to patients' desires and others comply with professional integrity, which rejects patients' desires in favor of their needs, as defined by the esoteric technical knowledge of the profession. Of course it is arrogant (and paternalistic) to presuppose too radical a distinction between what a patient can know about his or her condition and what a physician can know. (b) Another tension results from the demands of caring and those of scientific detachment. Caring is a cooperative, moral involvement while science is considered objective and noninvolved. (c) Stress also comes from patients' satisfaction with a physician and the fact of the physician's competence. Here again is the radical distinction between what a patient and a professional can judge. It depends upon accepting, in this case, a philosophic division between appearance and reality. The concept of professionalism would propose that the medical profession police those who get by on patient satisfaction alone and let those who are competent to practice compete for patient acceptance. In this circumstance, any pandering would at least have an Appollonian rather than a Pan-Dionysian base. (d) Finally, a fourth type of tension results when a physician's concern for the human person as a whole conflicts with another doctor's primary or exclusive concern with the human body. The first type of physician described in situations (a) and (d) seems to involve pathos and the second type pathology. Medical professionalism has, in its practice (rather than its preaching), tended to value knowledge and skill within the sphere of the pathologic and has disvalued knowledge and skill within the sphere of pathos.[36] This devaluation has led many nonphysicians to a philosophic attitude toward medicine that is consumeristic and contractual and emphasizes informed consent.[37] The arguments for this stance are very powerful. The trouble is that they fail to take account of what is implied in this essay: pathos is essential in medicine. There is little evidence, however, that those who argue for pathos know how to realize it. Unfortunately, too, there is little evidence that contemporary physicians (against whom this contractual model is framed) know how to realize pathos, either.

The implications of these states of ignorance are not favorable. Add to the need for pathos the incompatibility between pathos and the compelling contractual view, and add further the dearth of the arts of pathos, and the result is tragic in that there are two equally right but conflicting solutions to these problems. The rationality of a Sam Abelman conforms to the contractual view and seems morally right, but it alienates patients and fails. It *conflicts* with the desired and necesary magic of a Vogler, which symbolizes the second kind of solution. Yet, tragically, it is the nature of human existence that we want to respect as rational beings. That may be why the proper attitude is not to want to stop the swing of the pendulum that Dr. Marti-Ibanez mentions. Perhaps the best attitude is to become more humorous about it and to see more films.

APPENDIX
THE LAST ANGRY MAN

Sam Abelman, the physician in *The Last Angry Man*, is angry about the irrationality of his patients, the accelerating and unnecessary use of technology, the crimes in the ghetto, and the overly fancy machinery of the clinic. He is a man of action and integrity who looks like an older, more intense Albert Einstein. Sam loves to garden in the small backyard of his Brooklyn home. Indeed, he seems to worship nature; the writings of Thoreau serve him as a bible.

Practicing out of the home that he shares with his wife in a declining neighborhood, Sam does not make a good living. Most of his patients have moved away from the neighborhood, died, or sought less angry doctors. Thus, his patient load consists of lower-class people who are a source of frustration to him. Nevertheless, he treats them with belligerent dignity. For example, one poor, black juvenile delinquent, whom Sam places in the general category "galoot" (a label he uses very often), still receives gruff respect. Sam does not view such patients as wild animals; when they are patients, galoots are respected as humans. Thus, the gruffness is Sam's attempt to shout the delinquent into decent behavior, for Sam shouts out points, reasons, and arguments. His efforts with the delinquent are successful in a modest way, though the boy dies of a brain tumor.

The story begins with an advertising executive, Woody Trasher, noticing a brief newspaper story about Sam. Sam's nephew, an aspiring journalist, sent the story to the newspaper. Thrasher, like many in this story, may most aptly be characterized by clichés, partly because the story is a statement of ideals. Thus, Thrasher is a "hotshot," and he urgently needs an exciting idea for a television series in order to save his job and fancy income. The idea is for a series, entitled *Americans, U.S.A.*, that will show stories of valuable everyday people. Thrasher, in a desperate move, informs his employers of his idea for the series and claims that Sam has agreed to be first; he says this even before Sam has been contacted.

Much of the story displays Thrasher's character as he tries to woo Sam and manipulate Sam's few friends to secure Sam's participation. Some agree to help in exchange for Thrasher's supplying Sam with a modest house in a better neighborhood. Thrasher's superiors work this idea into the show as a surprise for the doctor.

As he observes Sam's life and anger, Thrasher comes to love Sam. When Sam finds out about the plan involving the house and refuses to do the show on that basis, Thrasher decides to defy his superiors; he respects Sam's pride by doing the show without the gift. But the whole broadcast is disrupted, first by Sam's being called to a police station in order to treat the ailing delinquent and then by Sam's suffering a massive heart attack as he is leaving the jail. Sam is brought home to die at age 68, having lived a fighting life—knowing that nothing of value comes easily. His model serves to help Thrasher become a better human being in Thrasher's own terms (to do the show for the viewers and for the doctor, not for himself), even as the delinquent had become better in his own terms.

Sam's demanding orientation to reality seems a cliché, too; it is a totally hard-nosed commitment to rational, selfless common sense. He wants to treat his patients as human, as whole persons, but without the slightest sensitivity to their fantasies or myths. These features of Sam are more accessible in the novel upon which the film is based, where, for example, Sam is humble enough, late in his career, to try to become a surgeon. He wants to be a surgeon because surgery is so clearly effective. So he studies surgery under a man who, as a child, observed in Sam's office.

This man, Heshy, becomes a master of anything he turns to, but as a technician with no soul, no warmth, he foretells why Sam is the *last* angry man. Heshy is in the new trend in medicine—remarkable technical mastery, group practice, clinic ownership and control. By contast, Sam, who at one time attempted suicide, knows what it is to suffer as a human being. But he cannot relate to patients at their primitive irrational level. His destructive but wise anger is intolerant of human frailties and human ties to the animal and natural world. He is a man of science. In the novel he rejects a career teaching exercise and nutrition, considering them less scientific. His insensitive demands on patients and rejection of their needs or desires for magic—including the new magic of technology—cause him to lose patients and fail to make an adequate living.

Sam is Janus-faced: he treats his patients as if they are or could be rational scientists about their problems; he treats his colleagues as if technology has come too far in replacing human interaction (no matter how argumentative) and clinical judgment with laboratory tests and the overreliance on machinery. The sketch of Sam, then, seems to be one in a series of characterizations of physicians—starting with Ibsen's Doctor Stockman[1]—who bravely stand alone, fighting for truth and decency, against galoots from below and self-serving technocrats from above.

Since he fights alone and constantly, by the end of his life Sam is worn out. Thus, the image of the quixotic Samuel Abelman fades at the same time that another image of the physician begins to intensify: that of the antisocial technical master who can work extraordinary feats of skill (one would never use the word "miracles" about such people). The fleshing out of this image occurs on the other side of the globe—in Korea in *M*A*S*H*.

*M*A*S*H*

Many of the central figures of *M*A*S*H* are made to appear likable. The story is set in a U.S. Army field hospital that seems to be ruled by a loudspeaker. As the film begins, the loudspeaker announces that a war film will be shown that night for the entertainment of the GIs. At the end of *M*A*S*H* the same loudspeaker tells us, "Tonight's movie has been *M*A*S*H*."

M*A*S*H is startling in its iconoclasm. Doctors are portrayed as crafty mechanics, desperately needed where they are because they are masters of a highly difficult and demanding technology. They exploit their power as technocrats and flaunt their disrepsect for the mores, morals, and authority of the broader world.

In M*A*S*H, the primary foils are some promilitary, prowar, fervent staff members—especially Dr. Burns and nurse (Major) Margaret Houlihan; the incompetent, unassertive commanding officer; the visiting self-indulgent maniacal general whose primary interests are sex with nurses and interhospital football games, which his group can win for high stakes; and the ineffectual Catholic priest.

The good guys, the antiheroes Hawkeye and Trapper, fail to conform to military protocol, including dress and courtesy. They get away with such misbehavior because their skills are needed and respected and would be lost if proper disciplinary procedures were initiated. Sometimes they get away with the improprieties because they actually use their skill as a physical force to achieve control of situations. For example, their prowess is so clear and so well known that they are ordered from Korea to Japan just to treat one congressman's son. By coincidence they meet an old friend of Hawkeye who is donating his skills to a Japanese children's hospital. He asks them to help save a baby and, as a favor to this friend—they apparently have no commitment to the baby—they agree. To do the operation, they must sneak into and use the military operating room. They get caught. To get off the legal hook, they anesthetize the commanding officer and take photographs of him with prostitutes. He drops all charges and the men return to Korea, where they go directly to the operating room and perform surgery in the outlandish, clownlike clothing they acquired for playing golf in Japan.

Not all of their wizardry is of this Robin Hood type. They sometimes use their medical power just to help themselves to certain things. For example, in a football game against the general's troops, they inject one of the opponents with a drug that makes him too goofy to play.

But the portrayal of the physicians as tacitly relying upon and exploiting their standing as masters of surgical arts pervades the film. They bait and humiliate a physician and nurse of higher rank, causing a psychotic breakdown in the physician, Major Burns. Burns is cast as a religious fanatic and as an incompetent surgeon—a combination that symbolizes the conflict between medicine or science and religion. Religion's defeat is clear in the way the priest is portrayed in the film.[2] For example, the quiet, shy, timid man awkwardly tries to welcome the new physicians by offering to help them with personal problems that may arise; nevertheless, he has to come to Hawkeye for the solution to a personal problem in the life of the oral surgeon. Still, as Dr. Major Burns shows, religion can apparently "ride on the coat tails" of an incompetent physician, who seemingly has to be psychotic in order to be religious. The mix of religiosity and medicine is too much for the good guys. They have to save medicine from the deplorable Dr. Burns. For although their personal behavior is wild, their medical acts are masterful. And, in being technocrats of the highest order, they can get away with their wild assaults and indulgences outside of surgery—even to the point of flagrant insubordination.

These physicians relate to their patients in a way altogether different from Abelman. Abelman would arm-wrestle a defiant patient if it were necessary to prove a point. He would badger to try to heal. But for whatever reasons, the doctors in *M*A*S*H* never speak to a patient. They are like craftsmen or engineers who have mastered the working of the most intricate machine—the human body. They hate the mad war and compensate for being trapped in it with warmongering companions by acting out—indulging in alcoholic and sexual debauchery, practical joking, and disrespect for authority.

In *M*A*S*H,* the misbehavior, the indulgence in what could be called "improper" or "unprofessional behavior," takes place in the area of life that is beyond the professional arena. The physicians are professional as such, but they are out of order as soldiers and (perhaps) as human beings as well. This is not true of the next film, where the healers' arena itself demands policing.

THE MAGICIAN

Bergman's *The Magician* is set in 1846 outside of Stockholm. At sunset, a coach bearing a sign for "Vogler's Magnetic Health Theatre" carries Vogler, who is the magician; Aman, who, though appearing to be a delicate man, is really Vogler's beautiful wife (named Manda); Granny, who is said to be hundreds of years old and one of the few true witches; Tubal, who seems to be barker for the troupe and often serves as spokesman for the mute magician; and Simson, the young driver. After riding through an eerie forest and assisting a dying actor, the troupe comes to a toll booth. Guards forcibly escort the group to a large, courtly building. There the troupe encounters the "host," Mr. Egerman; the chief of police, Mr. Starbeck; and the Royal Counselor on Medicine, Dr. Vergerus.

The stage is set for the struggle between doctor-scientist and magician. Although the film bills itself as a comedy, these are two humorless men who have large claim to what the healer should be. The magician works by symbolism and mesmerization. The doctor works by anatomical manipulation. Thus, they symbolize magician and technocrat, respectively.

The troupe has been summoned by the police chief's order at the request of the host and hostess, who say they have a great interest in the spiritual world—the world that, it would seem, is manipulated by true magicians. Tubal introduces Vogler as Mesmer's foremost student and declares, "The sickness which Mr. Volger cannot alleviate by his magnets is not yet known." But he adds, "Everything is completely scientific! Naturally." It evolves that this is quite the issue.

The townsmen know of the troupe and of its supranatural bent because the troupe ran a newspaper advertisment promising "sensational marvels, magic acts, health-giving magnets, and spine-tingling thrills of the senses."

The "mute" Vogler does not answer the probing questions of Vergerus, but Aman denies any healing powers on their part and any real magical power. He (she) insists that all they can do is trickery. Either interpretation of the troupe's activity—

mesmerism or trickery—is repugnant to the doctor. Tubal wants the painful confrontation to end. He boldly invites them to hold the troupe responsible if they have done anything unlawful. The police chief declares that this is what they intend to discover.

Just then Mrs. Egerman enters. Her child has died sometime earlier, and she wants to believe in soul and meaning but cannot. Her well-intentioned husband and his friends want her to side with them against the magician. They may believe that either choice would be a cure for her ills, but they seem to prefer that she become practical and choose to believe in nothing—at least nothing metaphysical. Upon her entry, Vergerus forces a seemingly painful and humiliating physical examination upon Vogler's speech organs. The enraged look of the magician occasions fear in Mrs. Egerman. Vergerus denies any physical evidence of the muteness. (He later turns out to have been right; Vogler is only feigning. Can this be a symbol for the lack of physical evidence for vital forces? Is Vergerus correct that there is no soul?) The challenge moves on. Vergerus demands that Vogler produce the advertised terrible visions in him. As Vogler seems to try, Vergerus speaks disinterestedly, denying that he hates the magician and avowing only an interest in doing an autopsy on him. Shortly, Vergerus seems to have a terrible vision, denies that he has, and suggests that he might regret not having had one. The official test of Vogler's skills is set for the next day.

In the morning, there are some apparently real magical events. Then Vogler is assaulted by an enraged servant who was a subject in one of the demonstrations. Vogler appears to have been killed in the attack, thus giving Vergerus his chance for the autopsy, anticipated in Vergerus's remarks the night before. It is actually performed upon the corpse of the actor who joined the troupe in the opening scene but, without even being known to the hosts, died during the night. In the midst of the secluded autopsy, the magician uses many tricks—some seem to be spiritual—to frighten Vergerus nearly to death. Later, the scientist regains some of his presence of mind and some of his power. He pretends to be totally unaffected, totally uninstructed by the fear. It looks as though the troupe will be run out of town (though there are some exchanges of places with some house staff), but, in a surprising triumph for the troupe, the king sends for them. The storm outside ceases and all ends happily.

NOTES

1. An earlier version of this paper was presented at the Popular Culture Association Conference in Pittsburgh, Pa., on April 28, 1970. I wish to thank Alex Bienkowski, Rabbi James Kessler, Drs. Anne Jones, Robert L. Jones, and James B. Speer, Jr., for their help and support with various drafts. In particular, I acknowledge the influence of Dr. Myron Zinn of San Antonio, Texas, who first sensitized me to the issues in *The Magician* and who continues to be a source of intellectual movement for me.

There are important objections to an essay like mine, which deals with contents alone. In the title essay of *Against Interpretation* (New York: Dell Publishing Co., 1966), Susan Sontag objects to taking the topics out of the context of an entire work of art as though the topics were shadows of real meaning or as though *experiencing* the whole work of art were too threatening and we had to tame being confronted by the art by reducing it to the level of rational understanding. She is explicit in warning against interpreting Bergman's work.

2. Novel: Gerald Greene, *The Last Angry Man* (New York: Pocket Books, 1974). Film: Daniel Mann, dir., *The Last Angry Man*, Columbia, 1959.

3. Novel: Richard Hooker, *M*A*S*H* (New York: Pocket Books, 1975). Film: Robert Altman, dir., *M*A*S*H*, Twentieth-Century Fox, 1971.

4. Ingmar Bergman, dir., *The Magician*, 1958. The screenplay can be found in *Four Screenplays of Ingmar Bergman* (New York: Simon & Schuster, 1960).

5. Stanley Hauerwas, *Vision and Virtue* (Notre Dame, Ind.: Fides Publications, 1974), chap. 4.

6. Susan Sontag, *On Photography* (New York: Farrar, Straus, and Giroux, 1973), pp. 153–61. Sontag is discussing photographic images in particular, but much of what she writes has application to film and even to nonvisual images.

7. Felix Marti-Ibanez, *The Patient's Progress* (New York: MD Publications, 1962), p. 124.

8. This now-classic distinction was forged by the nineteenth-century philosopher, Friedrich Nietzsche. For a full account of the evolution and place of this distinction in Nietzsche's thought, see Walter Kaufmann's *Nietzsche* (Princeton, N.J.: Princeton University Press, 1950).

9. Pan and Dionysus have been closely linked in the scholarly literature on mythology. See P. O. Morford and Robert J. Lenardon, *Classical Mythology* (New York: David McKay Co., 1972), p. 193. Carolyn Norris, "The Images of the Physician in Modern American Literature" (Ph.D. diss., University of Maryland, 1970), generated the categories of Priest (meaning technocratic) and Pan to synthesize the myriad of portrayals she had read. My characterizations are very much dependent upon hers. Further, see R. Seltzer's "The Exact Location of the Soul" and "The Surgeon As Priest," *Mortal Lessons* (New York: Touchstone Book, 1974) for a similar use of "priest" and the imagery to go with it. The reader might also be interested in the discussion by R. B. Scott in his "The Doctor in Contemporary Literature," *Lancet* 269 (1955): 341–43.

10. Adolf Guggenbuhl-Craig, *Power in the Healing Professions* (Zurich: Spring Publications, 1971), p. 103.

11. Carl Jung, "On the Psychology of the Trickster-Figure," *Four Archetypes*, trans R. F. C. Hull (Princeton, N.J.: Princeton University Press, 1959), p. 140.
12. Ibid., p. 144.
13. Ibid., pp. 136, 143.
14. Ibid., pp. 142, 146.
15. Ibid., p. 147.
16. I have found clarification and help in Philip Turner's unpublished "Ritual, Sickness and Death." Turner also relies upon the work of Victor Turner, including *Schism and Continuity in an African Society* (Manchester, England: Manchester University Press, 1957); *Ndembu Divination: Its Symbolism and Technique*, Rhodes Livingston Papers, No. 31 (Manchester, England: Manchester University Press, 1961); *Chihamba, The White Spirit*, Rhodes Livingston Papers, No. 33 (Manchester, England: Manchester University Press, 1962); "Three Symbols of Passages in Ndembu Circumcision Ritual," *Essays in the Ritual of Social Relations*, ed. Max Gluckman (Manchester, England: Manchester University Press, 1962); *The Forest of Symbols* (Ithaca, N.Y.: Cornell University Press, 1967); *The Drums of Affliction* (Oxford: At the University Press, 1968); *The Ritual Process: Structure and Anti-Structure* (Chicago: Aldine Press, 1969). Philip Turner also acknowledges insight from Mary Douglas's *Natural Symbols* (New York: Vintage Books, 1970).
17. See Owsei Temkin, "Materialism in French and German Physiology of the Early 19th Century," *Bulletin of the History of Medicine* 20 (1946): 322–27. It is ironic, though, that Mesmer himself started on the scientific side of the divide. H. Ellenberger writes: "The emergence of dynamic psychiatry can be traced to the year 1775, to a clash between the physician Mesmer and the exorcist Gassner"—quoted by E. M. Scott in "Combining the Roles of 'Priest' and 'Physician': A Clinical Case," *Journal of Religion and Health* 18 (1979): 160.
18. Antics may be a kind of ritual. Cf. the discussion of jokes by Mary Douglas cited below in note 32.
19. See June Goodfield, "Humanity in Science: A Perspective and a Plea," *Science* 198 (1977): 580.
20. See Alan Thornhill, "Drama As A Therapeutic Force," *Medicine, Morals and Man*, ed. Ernest Claxton and H. A. C. McKay (London: Blandford Press, 1969).
21. Mel Gussow, "The Time of the Wounded Hero," *The New York Times*, 15 April 1979, pp. 1, 30.
22. Rudolph Virchow, *Disease, Life and Man: Selected Essays*, trans. Lelland J. Rather (Stanford, Calif.: Stanford University Press, 1958), p. 57.
23. See Darrel W. Amundsen, "Images of a Physician in Classical Times," *Journal of Popular Culture* 11 (1978): 642–55; see also Amundsen's "Romanticizing the Ancient Medical Profession: The Characterization of the Physician in the Graeco-Roman Novel," *Bulletin of the History of Medicine* 48 (1974): 320–37; George W. Corner, "Medicine in the Modern Drama," *Annals of Medical History* N.S. 10 (1938): 309–17; Jessie Dodson, "Doctors in Literature," *Library Association Record* 71 (1969): 269–74; Christine E. Petersen, *The Doctors in French Drama, 1700–1775* (New York: Columbia University Press, 1938), pp. 4–7.
24. Joseph Campbell, *The Hero With a Thousand Faces* (New York: Pantheon Books, 1949), p. 9. Of course, there are godlike heroes who control destiny; tragic heroes who try to control destiny and fail; and comic heroes who, controlled by destiny, succeed in mundane attempts. Antiheroes, who operate outside of a destiny, do not seem to try to do very much.
25. Here I was influenced by S. Hauerwas's *Truthfulness and Tragedy* (Notre Dame, Ind.: University of Notre Dame Press, 1977), esp. chap. 14. See also p. 195.

26. Virchow, *Disease, Life and Man,* pp. 205–6.

27. For a recent promagic plea, see "A Symbolic Triangle: Hippocrates, Psyche and Pandora" by Bernard V. Dryer, published by the Society for Health and Human Values. Sociologists have suggested that nurses take up something akin to what I might call the magical burden of doctors. See, for example, Fred E. Katz, "Nurses," in *The Semi-Professions and their Organization,* ed. A. Etzioni (New York: Free Press, 1969), especially pp. 56, 65–66.

28. Jung, "On the Psychology of the Trickster-figure," pp. 144, 147–48, 151–52.

29. S. Cavell, "What Becomes of Things on Film?", *Philosophy and Literature* 2 (1978): 251.

30. C. Hyers, *Zen and the Comic Spirit* (Philadelphia: Westminister, 1974).

31. Mary Douglas, "Social Control of Cognition: Some Factors in Joke Perception," *Man* N.S. 3 (1968): 364.

32. Ibid., p. 365.

33. See, e.g., Lewis Thomas's sarcastic critique, "On Magic in Medicine," *The New England Journal of Medicine* 297 (1978): 461–63. This is not to deny the inordinate harm done by false magic. For an account of this, see J. H. Young's *The Medical Messiahs* (Princeton, N.J.: Princeton University Press, 1967).

34. See Norman Cousins, "Anatomy of An Illness (As Perceived by the Patient)," *The New England Journal of Medicine* 295 (1976): 1458–63; Raymond A. Moody, Jr., *Laugh After Laugh* (Jacksonville, Fla.: Headwaters Press, 1978).

35. Eliot Friedson, *The Profession of Medicine* (New York: Harper and Row, 1970).

36. The major exception to this is the paternalistic deceptions which experienced doctors often perpetrate because they believe in a close mind-body-connection or because they care to avoid the purely mental distress they expect from telling unhappy truths.

37. See Eleanor Glass, "Restructuring Informed Consent: Legal Therapy for the Doctor-Patient Relationship," *Yale Law Journal* 79 (1970): 1533–76, for a statement of the contractual model as a replacement for the pathos of the good old doctor-patient relationship. Note that Glass's paper is relatively early in the new wave of external attention to medicine. Also see a classic statement of the options available for structuring the doctor-patient relationship in Robert M. Veatch, "Models for Ethical Medicine in a Revolutionary Age," *Hastings Center Reports* 2 (1972): 5–7.

Appendix

1. Henrik Ibsen, *Enemy of the People,* in *Four Major Plays,* trans. Rolf Fjeld. 2 vols. (New York: New American Library, 1970). I am indebted to "The Doctor As Dramatic Hero" by D. Heyward Brock (read at the Popular Culture Association Conference in Pittsburgh on April 28, 1979) for some of the points about the history of the use of doctors in literature.

2. In the novel, the priest is recognized as a significant individual who even possessed healing powers. It is interesting (startling) to compare the portrayal of the priest in *M*A*S*H** with the representation of Father Francis P. Duffy in *The Fighting 69th* (1941), directed by William Keighley.

Humpty Dumpty: A Literary Challenge to the Concept of Personality Integration

KATHRYN ALLEN RABUZZI

State University of New York Upstate Medical Center

> Humpty Dumpty sat on a wall,
> Humpty Dumpty had a great fall.
> All the King's horses, and all the
> King's men,
> Couldn't put Humpty Dumpty
> together again.

While this rhyme, like all of Mother Goose, is often construed politically, it also presents an image of human fragility. In today's vernacular, Humpty Dumpty "had it all together" until he became "spaced out." Seemingly, current slang says much the same about human personality as traditional jingles do. But a closer look at both suggests that they reflect radically different assumptions. Humpty Dumpty, after all, was at one time a unified entity. By contrast, most youth who speak of "getting it all together" sound as if that were a barely possible ideal that few can achieve. Like Adam and Eve, Humpty Dumpty fell from an original wholeness, but like questers everywhere, seekers hoping to "get it all together" search for a condition not yet attained. The difference between these two points of departure is crucial to a clear understanding of what "getting it all together," or personality integration, means to our age.

One may legitimately question whether Humpty Dumpty ranks as literature or not, but true literature functions typically as a *speculum mentis,* a mirror of humanity. Consequently, we can look to it for fairly accurate reflections of ourselves as human beings at various stages in time. Although we may take for granted that personality refers to something stable and substantive, the derivation of the word from the Latin *persona,* meaning mask, immediately suggests a discontinuity between it and its "wearer." If that is so, the notion of stability immediately becomes questionable: Why only one mask and not many? Why do we automatically correlate the mask with personality rather than the process of masking? If the process is primary, what does that mean for our concept of personality integration? Most crucial of all the questions: Does personality integration necessarily mean putting all the masks, or parts, in one package?

To focus attention on these issues, I draw from literature some representative examples to indicate how concepts of human personality and personality development have evolved over time. Three of the stories I examine are traditional in both form and content, reflecting in order primitive, religious, and modern humanity. The last two examples both reflect postmodern humanity, one through altered form, the other through new content. While such a typology is obviously broad and schematic, it is intended to indicate general directions in human evolution and to suggest that the idea that humans either can or should try to "get it all together" may no longer be appropriate to our era.

The first literary image of human personality I want to consider is Trickster, a figure found in various forms throughout the world. He appears, for example, in tales from China, Japan, the Near East, and ancient Greece. Furthermore, Trickster belongs to one of the oldest known myths, making him a vulnerable mirror of humanity's earliest attempts to envision itself and the world into which it is thrown. The particular Trickster image I wish to examine is drawn from the Winnebago Indian Trickster cycle, which presents him as an imprecisely proportioned, shapeless creature. So little self-awareness does he possess that he scarcely realizes his separation from his surroundings. Like a very young infant, he neither knows his sexual identity nor understands where he himself leaves off and the external world begins. Probably the best-known tale of this cycle is one entitled "Trickster Burns Anus and Eats His Own Intestines,"[1] in which he grabs some birds for food, and before eating them, reminds himself that cooking them is what a man does. Thus, within the story, he overtly reminds himself what behavior is appropriate to humanity. Throughout the story he talks to himself, much like a very small child, telling himself what he must do: while waiting for the meat to cook, he should sleep, but in order to protect his dinner from thieves, he must leave it guarded. Speaking now to his anus, whom he addresses as "younger brother," he admonishes it to keep watch while he sleeps. Rather predictably, his anus cannot prevent the theft of the two roasting ducks. When Trickster awakens, his anger is so intense that he chastizes his anus by burning it over the fire. Only slowly, as Trickster feels the pain, does he make the connection that he and his anus form part of the same human being.

Trickster, obviously, is a figure who reflects the process whereby humans originally learned to become human. The major emphases in all the tales of this cycle focus upon distinguishing self from other entities, both animate and inanimate, discriminating female from male, recognizing the boundaries of self, and distinguishing humanity from animality. Although human infants must also learn to make these discriminations for themselves, unlike Trickster and the primitive humans who conceived him, they do so within a context generated by years of cultural acceptance that we are not animals, objects, androgynes, nor brothers to our body-parts.

By contrast with the cloudy understanding of personality differentiation present in this story, at a considerably advanced stage of human evolution, humanity looks not to distinguish itself from the animals that seem so much like it, but rather it now seeks to identify with a wholly different realm: the gods above. Thus, for example, in early Greek myths we find an intermingling of gods and humans and, at the same time, the development of godlike men called heroes. Within the Judeo-Christian tradition this impulse culminates in the figure of Christ. Although the Christ story is too familiar to require much reiteration, it is perhaps helpful to recall that Christ was not, according to official doctrine, originally human. He was, after all, as the Son of God, originally deity itself, choosing freely to become human through kenosis, a process in which divinity empties itself out to allow human nature to replace it. Thus, in Christ we see an image of being directly opposite to that depicted by Trickster. Whereas Trickster reflects the lower animal becoming something higher through human differentiation, Christ reflects something higher, the divine, becoming lower, or human. By juxtaposing the two stories, we can see two distinct stages in human understanding of limitation and separation: on the one hand, humans are distinct from the animals; on the other, from the gods. Jesus remained a model of human being for much of the world for more than 1,500 years, and is so today for many individuals. Whereas the primitive Trickster tales reflect human being slowly coming to awareness of itself as distinct from its surroundings, the story of Christ indicates an orientation in which human awareness is directed towards an ideal—both an ideal world and an ideal image of humanity in the person of Christ. As such, it is an image impossible of literal replication.

Inevitably, as human society altered historically, this older religious ideal slowly yielded to a predominantly secular orientation in which, as Pope put it, "The proper study of mankind is man." In this period, beginning roughly with the Renaissance and lasting to some extent through our own day, but beginning to change from about 1850 to 1900 on, literature altered its previous emphasis on saints' tales, legends, exempla, and romances to new, secular stories, plays and poems that culminated eventually in the novel. Particularly relevant to understanding personality integration is the *bildungsroman,* the novel of apprenticeship or initiation. Typical of this broad category is J. D. Salinger's *Catcher in the Rye,* in which the young protagonist, Holden Caulfield, finds himself repeatedly unable to adjust to his environment. Kicked out of one prep school after another, Holden tells his story to an unseen psychiatrist, focusing primarily on his final day at Pency Prep and his subsequent journey home to see his younger sister Phoebe, the only fully positive image of humanity in Holden's life. Like many American novels, Holden's story is a quest for an ideal promised land. As is typical of all *bildungsromanen, Catcher* involves an initiation into the adult world. For Holden that initiation involves painfully extended confrontations with various forms of adult phoniness. Gone for Holden is the older religious imagery, which allows for the actuality of some promised land to come. In Holden's ideal world he would like to be a catcher in the rye, by which he means that he would stand in an extensive field of rye, waiting to catch all the little kids he envisions tumbling into it from the cliff above.

Yet this is no romance, and Holden ends up in his psychiatrist's office, telling his tale, its eventual outcome unresolved.

In his case the issue of personality integration involves a choice between perpetual childhood, which, carried over into adulthood, is labeled differentness, deviation, or even craziness, or adaptation to the pretenses of adult life. No other choice exists within the framework of the story.

Such choices, which until recently seemed to be the only ones available to individuals within our society, given the assumptions of psychoanalysis and related therapies, appear to many a dead end. Nonetheless, for others who came of age within the twentieth century, the *bildungsroman,* regardless of its particular content, remains the image of what a novel is supposed to be. By implication, its characters, likewise, represent what human personality should be. Meanwhile, however, new forms of literature have arisen that no longer fit the familiar modes. Words like *antihero* and *antinovel,* for example, are now commonplace in literary criticism. Although from the time of the Romantics on, the ideas of literature have frequently been designed to *épater les bourgeoisie,* to shock the middle class, and reject accepted ways of thinking, formal changes such as those characteristic of the twentieth century did not really become marked until after World War II. Writers like James Joyce, T. S. Eliot, William Faulkner, and Ernest Hemingway, though obviously major innovators, still present recognizably human personalities operating under the assumption that there is such a thing as human nature. By contrast, writers in the tradition of the Absurd, stemming from mime, commedia dell'arte, Shakespeare's clowns, vaudeville, Dada, and German Expressionism, present images of humanity that seem totally at variance with older conceptions. In this category fall numerous dramatists including Samuel Beckett, Eugene Ionesco, Arthur Adamov, and Harold Pinter. Then there are the surrealist poets like André Breton and Guillaume Appollinaire and the novelists of black humor like Nathaneal West and Flannery O'Connor. And finally there are the so-called metafictionists like John Barthes or William Gass.

Though differing in many ways, all these writers have in common a dissolution of language and/or form that marks them off from their predecessors more thoroughly perhaps than any of their earlier iconoclastic counterparts. This break signals a discontinuity in human personality as radical as that depicted in the tales of Trickster, suggesting that we, postmodern humanity, stand on the verge of changes as momentous to human consciousness as those Trickster must have experienced at the other end of the scale as he came to know what it meant to be human.

To gain some understanding of this shift, I wish to focus on some of Samuel Beckett's characters. In all his work, whether his plays, poems, novels, or short stories, Beckett continuously frustrates expectations. He repeatedly conjoins and disjoins things temporal and spatial so that he violates two of our strongest presuppostions concerning personality: first, he opens up the whole question of whether there is such a possibility as continuity of self in time, and second, he raises the issue of whether two entities existing simultaneously in time are, in fact, spatially distinct. Thus, the characters he presents seem almost to be counterparts to the primitive Trickster.

In his *Stories and Texts for Nothing*, for example, Beckett's speaker is a nameless "I" who negates the seemingly unquestionable identity we ordinarily assume exists between "I" and "me" by saying "if I were me." Furthermore, Beckett does not limit himself merely to disjoining the subjective and objective halves of the first person; he also questions the concepts of person and number by shifting his speaker periodically and without warning into "we," "it," "him," "they," and "you." In all cases the speaker is referring to himself, assuming one can still legitimately use that expression. Thus Beckett radically questions the existence of a stable identity for his endlessly speaking persona. Yet the reader nonetheless considers the speaker in all thirteen texts and all three stories not as sixteen separate speakers but as a single person. This paradox reflects Beckett's frequently expressed idea that persons are both "the same, yet another," a theme he varies endlessly throughout his corpus. Obviously Beckett refers to such persons, if such they be, on two different levels at a time. On the level of physical appearance, a Beckett personality looks sufficiently the same from one encounter to the next to enable a perceiver to recognize him. Yet, as Beckett repeatedly indicates, no entity existing in time is *ever* the same from one moment to the next. Thus, for example, in act 2 of *Waiting for Godot*, Vladimir and Pozzo have the following exchange:

Vladimir: And you are Pozzo?
Pozzo: Certainly I am Pozzo.
Vladimir: The same as yesterday?

Pozzo: Yesterday?
Vladimir: We met yesterday. Do you not remember?
Pozzo: I don't remember having met anyone yesterday. But tomorrow I won't remember having met anyone today.

Beckett thus leaves the reader wondering whether two spatially separate Pozzos exist. Or has time so altered a single Pozzo that yesterday is unconnected from today, making it nonexistent for him? In the latter situation Pozzo would clearly represent what we normally consider to be a nonintegrated personality. In fact, he and all the countless Beckett characters who so closely resemble him in this respect, very much mimic the symptoms of a schizophrenic whom psychoanalyst Eugene Minkowski describes. Explaining his patient's lack of what we consider normal time sense, Minkowski writes:

> . . . each day kept an unusual independence, failing to be immersed in the perception of any life continuity; each day life began anew, like a solitary island in a gray sea of passing time. . . . every day was an exasperating monotony of the same words, the same complaints, until one felt that this being had lost all sense of necessary continuity. Such was the march of time for him.[2]

Now if Beckett were an exception, it would be logical to ask if he were not also schizophrenic. But he is no exception. All the Absurdists in one way or another question the validity of assuming a single integrated self. In Simon Gray's *Otherwise Engaged,* for example, Hinch, the main character, is so disengaged from life that he remembers nothing: for him life is such a series of discrete and continuously new moments that he fails to recall who his closest friend's ex-wife was. Nor can he remember within the space of a single day what most closely concerns his only brother. Is Hinch a person as we traditionally comprehend the term? More precisely, does he possess an integrated personality?

Even if one dismisses the dramatists of the Absurd as aberrations, there is further evidence of prevalent personality disintegration from other types of contemporary literature. Whereas the Absurdists tend to dissolve form as well as personality, science fiction writers typically do only the latter. To pick a single example from this genre, Ursula Le Guin, in her brilliant novel, *The Lathe of Heaven,* presents a protagonist who dreams what he calls effective dreams: they literally change the world.

As the story opens, protagonist George Orr is consulting a psychiatrist who predictably assumes his new patient is schizophrenic. Repeatedly, within the story Orr dreams effectively so that he endlessly recreates the world and all its surviving inhabitants with tiny, mindboggling variations. Consequently, aside from Orr and eventually his psychiatrist, no one in the world possesses what we would ordinarily define as a temporally integrated personality.

Are such plays and stories simply coincidental freaks? If Ezra Pound is correct that "poets are the antennae of the human race," then the prominence of such anomic characters in modern literature suggests we are witnessing a human metamorphosis of evolutionary significance. Increasingly, not only the arts, but psychiatric theory such as that of R. D. Laing or Thomas Szasz, for example, communicates new visions of human selfhood. As psychologist Kenneth Gergen suggests, "getting it all together" into a single self may not even be desirable.[3] Though the notion that personality should be integrated seems axiomatic, that concept may already be a relic of an earlier mode of human being. In an age that futurologist Alvin Toffler characterizes as containing "too much change, too soon," personality integration might conceivably be maladaptive behavior. If so, the frequent cry of the young to "get it all together" may already symbolize a vanished "golden age" that all the King's horses and all the King's men cannot put back together again.

NOTES

1. Paul Radin, *The Trickster* (New York: Philosophical Library, 1956).
2. Eugene Minkowski, "Findings in a Case of Schizophrenic Depression," trans. Barbara Bliss, in *Existence,* ed. Rollo May, Ernest Angel, and Henri F. Ellenberger (New York: Simon and Schuster, 1958), p. 133.
3. Kenneth Gergen, "Multiple Identity: The Healthy, Happy Human Being Wears Many Masks," *Psychology Today* 5 (1972).

Notes on Contributors

DENNIS G. CARLSON, associate professor at the Johns Hopkins School of Hygiene and Public Health in the Department of International Health, directs the Program in the Humanities and Public Health at Johns Hopkins University. Having received advanced degrees in medicine, behavioral science, and the history of medicine, Carlson has published in the *Royal Society of Health Journal, The Ethiopia Medical Journal,* and *Bulletin of the History of Medicine.*

WILMER J. COGGINS is dean of the College of Community Health Sciences and associate dean of the University of Alabama School of Medicine. Active in many medical organizations, Coggins has published in *The New England Journal of Medical Education, The Journal of Family Practice,* and the *Annals of the New York Academy of Sciences.*

EDMUND L. ERDE, contributor of articles on free will and determinism and the philosophy of medicine to the *Encyclopedia of Bioethics,* is associate professor of the Philosophy of Medicine at the College of Medicine and Dentistry of New Jersey, New Jersey School of Osteopathic Medicine, Camden. The author of a variety of journal articles and invited papers, Erde has also conducted workshops and seminars on philosophical and ethical perspectives of health care.

PETER WILLIAM GRAHAM has published articles in the *Journal of the History of Medicine and Allied Sciences, Interdisciplinary Perspectives, Literature and Medicine, Perspectives in Biology and Medicine,* and *Encyclopedia of Short Fiction.* Graham is assistant professor in the Department of English at Virginia Polytechnic Institute and State University.

MICHAEL S. GREGORY, professor of English at San Francisco

State University, is program director for the National Endowment for the Humanities-funded development grant, "Science and Humanities: a Program for Convergence," known as the NEXA Program. He also directs a project funded by the Mellon Foundation to disseminate the NEXA Program to other California state university and college campuses. Gregory is active as a consultant, reviewer, and panelist for NEH and NSF, and his publications and presentations reflect his research and interest in humanities and science.

VAN RENSSELAER POTTER, the recipient of many distinguished international honors, is professor of Oncology at the University of Wisconsin and former assistant director of the McArdle Laboratory for Cancer Research at the University of Wisconsin Medical School. The author of many publications on biochemistry, cancer research, and subjects related to environmental bioethics, Potter has written a textbook, *Bioethics: Bridge to the Future,* that presents an interdisciplinary approach to biological problems facing man.

KATHRYN ALLEN RABUZZI is a research associate in Humanities and Medicine at the Upstate Medical Center, Syracuse, New York. The author of publications concentrating on religion and English, Rabuzzi is the editor of the annual journal *Literature and Medicine.* Her most recent book is *The Sacred and the Feminine: Toward a Theology of Housework.*

MICHAEL E. RUSE, professor of Philosophy at the University of Guelph, has published in many journals in the areas of history and philosophy of biology, the history and philosophy of science, and ethical questions in biology and medicine. His major books include *Sociobiology: Sense or Nonsense?, The Philosophy of Biology,* and *The Darwinian Revolution: Science Red in Tooth and Claw.*

DAVID C. THOMASMA is director of the Medical Humanities Program at Loyola University Stritch School of Medicine. During his term directing the Human Values and Ethics Program of the Center for Health Sciences at the University of Tennessee, Professor Thomasma was project director of five grants relating medicine and humanities. Author of numerous articles on philosophy of science, philosophy of medicine, and technology and culture, he has also authored, with E. D. Pellegrino, *A Philosophical Basis of Medical Practice.*

JAMES E. TROSKO is professor of Human Development in the College of Human Medicine at Michigan State University. He has received various research grants and career development awards from the National Cancer Institute at the National Institute of Health, and his recent publications have appeared in journals such as *Advances in Radiology, Cancer Research, Quarterly Review of Biophysics,* and *Science.* In 1979 Trosko received the United Kingdom-Environmental Mutagen Society's "Serle" Award for pioneering research on DNA in mammalian cells.

RICHARD M. ZANER is the Anne Geddes Stahlman Professor in Medical Ethics at Vanderbilt University. An active participant in many professional organizations, Zaner serves on the editorial board of numerous philosophical journals and is general editor of *Selected Studies in Phenomenology and Existential Philosophy.* His most recent book is *The Context of Self: A Phenomenological Inquiry Using Medicine As A Clue.*

Index